ACUPUNCTURE THERAPY

An abridged and revised edition of the first
comprehensive textbook of Chinese acupuncture in the
English by a founder member of the British College
of Acupuncture.

ACUPUNCTURE THERAPY

The Philosophy, Principles and Methods of Chinese Acupuncture

by

Dr Mary Austin

Illustrations by
Denis Lawson-Wood

TURNSTONE PRESS LIMITED
Wellingborough, Northamptonshire

First published 1974
First paperback Edition 1981

© ASI PUBLISHERS INC. 1972, 1981

British Library Cataloguing in Publication Data

Austin, Mary, *b. 1914*
   Acupuncture therapy.
   1. Acupuncture
   I. Title
   615'.892   RN184

   ISBN 0-85500-142-9

Printed in Great Britain by
Nene Litho, Earls Barton, Northamptonshire
and bound by
Weatherby Woolnough, Wellingborough, Northamptonshire.

Contents

List of major illustrations

ILLUSTRATION SYMBOLS

▲ = Forbidden to Moxa
■ = Forbidden to Needle
✕ = Forbidden to Needle and Moxa
✱ = Forbidden to Moxa for children under 7 years of age
† = Avoid piquing if possible, extremely painful
φ = Forbidden to pique during pregnancy

Preface

Since this work first appeared in 1972, there has been tremendous growth in the practice of acupuncture in the Western world. Many schools, colleges and clinics have been set up, and all are flourishing. The fact that it has become acceptable to seek acupuncture treatment must be seen as evidence of its efficacy in relieving health problems.

Acupuncture should not be regarded as a cure for any condition; it is not a panacea. What it can often do is to relieve acute symptoms so that the body's need for balance can be facilitated.

My hope is that acupuncture will find its natural place in the field of medicine. It is best used as a preventative treatment to help reduce the present over-dependence on drugs. If regular 'check-ups' were made, illnesses could be averted through recognition that one of the body's systems is weakening.

Since this book first appeared, I have been twice the guest of the People's Republic of China, to see the evidence of their ancient acupuncture skills, and I witnessed many successful treatments for every type of problem. During my second visit in 1979 I saw the new technique of electrical acupuncture without the use of needles. When I trained, I learned the ancient method of inserting needles by hand, and infusing my thoughts, my own energy and love to assist the healing process.

This paperback edition has been produced for easy reference by students of natural therapies. The repertories and test papers have been omitted; otherwise the material is the same as the hardcover edition.

'Knowledge with Wisdom is what the World is seeking.' (Chinese proverb)

Mary Austin
London, 1980

Introduction

This textbook has been prepared with the utmost care in order to put before you, systematically, all the necessary basic information to enable you to study and understand Acupuncture.

From time to time I shall suggest various 'dodges' to aid memorizing; in general, however, you can rely upon this — the more avenues through which information goes into your head, the more rapidly and firmly will it become established there. Use as many senses as you can — so that the information goes in through your eyes, your ears, and through your touch-sense. There will be occasions when it can also go in through your senses of taste and smell.

For example: in order to memorize a group of facts such as The Path of a Meridian, Its Number, The Organ associated with it, The Associated Element, Associations with that Element, such as 'flavour', 'colour', 'time of day', 'season of the year', etc., proceed as follows:—

Read the information out loud;

Trace the path of the Meridian with your finger, or at least touch the first and last points of the Path;

Look at the appropriate chart or diagram, touch it.

If it is significant to remember 'Salty Flavour' then actually place a grain or two of salt on the tip of your tongue.

Look at an example of the 'Colour'.

If you do these things you will be quite pleasantly surprised to find just how quickly something learned in this way goes in — and goes in for good — with relatively little effort. I am confident of this.

Be patient and proceed with caution, especially when it comes to trying things out in actual clinical experiment. There some acupuncture points which may be treated with safety in almost any condition or circumstance — experiment with these first. There are some ''Forbidden Points''—these will have to be memorized in order to avoid accidents or mistakes.

The Acupuncture ''Needle Techniques'' are purposely postponed until late in this text. This helps the student by not offering him too early the temptation to ''try sticking a needle in'' before he is sufficiently aware of what he is doing.

Nevertheless you will, very early in the book, have a treatment technique explained to you other than the 'needle'. Thus you will soon be able to put what you have learned to practical use *without any risk of accidents with needles.*

Part one

THE ORGAN MERIDIANS AND THE TWELVE PULSES OF ACUPUNCTURE

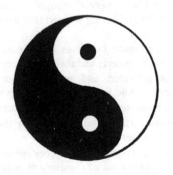

1

Yin-Yang: The Bi-polar Energy of the Body

When we begin our study of Acupuncture it is of the utmost importance for us to realize that the acupuncture orientation is quite different from that of any accepted Western medical approach. Though Western medical knowledge may be of advantage to the student in some respects, it may also be a disadvantage in others. It will be an actual hindrance to the student to the extent that he has already become conditioned in, and prejudiced in favour of, the Western notions.

We shall need to grasp thoroughly just what it is that treatment at Acupuncture points aims to achieve. What exactly is it that the Acupuncture practitioner tries to influence, alter, stimulate, sedate, and so on?

We cannot use Acupuncture with any worthwhile degree of efficiency or confidence unless we not only understand what forces we are manipulating or dealing with but also have a firm foundation knowledge of Acupuncture anatomy. This means that we must know, very thoroughly, exactly where to find the Acupuncture points on the body. Having learned this we then need to know what to do at the points, and when.

Our very first task is to make ourselves acquainted with a brief but comprehensive survey of the basic concepts and theory of Acupuncture.

The Life-process is activated and maintained by what is called, in Acupuncture, Vital Force or Life Energy. This energy is derived from our environment through such processes as respiration and nutrition, is converted into assimilable form by certain organs and is stored in the body and distributed throughout the system by other organs.

We, in Acupuncture, accept it as a basic concept or premise that this Vital Force (Life Energy) is a manifestation of a unitary bi-polar energy that, in living creatures, permeates every cell and tissue of the organism—in form, structure and process.

The behaviour of this Life Force, e.g. its rhythm, periodicity, polar equilibrium, polarization and depolarization, etc., constitutes the Laws of Nature.

For every mode or form of existence, from the largest system or organization to the minutest individual system (macroscopic to microscopic) there is an appropriate normal behaviour pattern or complex of natural laws that must be observed. There is no escaping the absolute imperative of Natural Law.

The working of Life Force may be considered as in three phases: the bringing into existence or ''birth''; the maintaining of existence in the space-time world or ''living''; and the taking out of existence or ''death''.

The birth or creation of anything represents a particular manifestation of the predominance of the positive, organizing or focussing polarity of Life Energy. This polarity is called Yang.

Death, destruction, or taking out of existence, represents the predominant or triumphal activity of the negative, dis-organizing or dispersing polarity of Life Energy. This polarity is called Yin.

Between the two extremes of birth and death there occurs some sort of continuum, or series of rhythms, dynamic balancings and un-balancings, creations of tension and relaxations of tension, cycles of predominance of Yin or of Yang, etc., the totality of which (in any organism) represents that organism's life span.

Yin and Yang, two Chinese words, are the only two Chinese words I shall constantly be using — I may from time to time mention some other Chinese name or word, but only in passing, not for you to remember. But ''Yin'' and ''Yang'' you must make part of your own habitual vocabulary.

At this point let us be quite clear: activity Yang and activity Yin are not two separate or different forces, but represent polarities of the one force, the life force or vital energy.

A human being represents a complex aggregate of polar tensions and relaxations, processes, rhythms, and so on; and a human being is said to be in health when all the appropriate rhythmic processes, dynamic balances, etc., occur appropriately for the fulfilment of the normal or natural human life span.

Life force never changes its unitary nature, but it is forever in a continuous state of change of polarity predominance.

Any disturbance of natural or proper balance which, if allowed to go on and is not restored to what it should be, would tend to shorten the normal life span represents a state of ill-health, sickness, disease, etc. The disturbance or im-balance may be quite small, so small as to be undetectable through any outward symptoms; or it may be a gross disturbance manifesting in quite distressing and horrible symptoms.

In Acupuncture we recognize that any disease has two main phases (i) an invisible and (ii) a visible. The first phase represents an energy imbalance or disturbance or weakness before it has shown itself in the body tissues or processes as organic or other symptoms in process, structure or function detectable out-wardly, visibly.

The highest art of the Acupuncture practitioner is in the becoming aware of a first stage disturbance or potential sickness before it has become gross — and treating the disturbance at that first stage effectively to forestall or prevent the disease from actually happening. This preventive aspect of Acupuncture therapy will be considered later on in this text.

The second phase of a disturbed energy balance occurs when the unchecked first stage imbalance begins to manifest in gross, outward symptoms. It is, alas,

with this second stage that most of the work of a Western Acupuncture practitioner will be — for, at the present day, patients do not come to a practitioner
until they are overtly ill.

An acupuncteur, then, first aims to locate the energy imbalance and
ascertain its nature. Having done this he aims to restore the balance to what it
should be normally by manipulating the vital energy.

The practitioner thinks and works in terms of vital energy rhythms, polar
changes, restoration of proper balance at deep levels. He never, never aims to
suppress symptoms — he considers source not end-product.

This brings us to the question: Where is it possible to influence polar imbalances with predictable precision through manipulation of vital energy? This is
the topic for the following section.

The Meridians (or Pathways) of Energy

Bearing in mind that the vital energy (circulating throughout the human
organism) is transformed, generated in, and stored and distributed by internal
organs, we realize that the paths of the energy circulation in and among the organs
themselves cannot be acted upon directly. This inner circulation we can call 'the
Core Circulation'. The energy cycles belonging to this Core Circulation will come
under consideration later in the course, when we study the Five Elements and the
laws governing the manipulation of energy.

Vital energy permeates every living cell and tissue; this naturally must
include the surface or near-surface tissues. The circulation of this surface energy
follows well established paths. These pathways form a definite pattern of lines
known in Acupuncture as the Meridians. The circulation of energy in the
Meridians we refer to as 'the Peripheral Circulation'.

The Core Circulation and the Peripheral Circulation are linked by numerous
internal pathways which, all together, we call the 'Mediate Circulation'.

Vital energy can be manipulated only where we can reach it — this clearly is
on or near the surface.

Observation, experience, and experiment over many thousands of years (by
Far-Eastern practitioners) have resulted in the recognition of numerous locations,
on or near the skin, where vital energy can be predictably influenced by
manipulation, and thus whereat energy imbalances, deficiencies, excesses,
blockages and escapes can be restored to normal. It is these peripheral circulation
points or Meridian points that we, in Acupuncture, must learn and be able to
locate exactly. These points on the skin are those known as Acupuncture Points.

There are some surface points used in Acupuncture that are not on the
Meridians. You should be aware of this, but we shall not be dealing with them.
Our concern is with the points on the Meridians—and if you know these, and are
able to use them properly, you will have all the essentials of a good practitioner at
your finger-tips.

The elementary anatomy of Acupuncture, then, consists of the knowledge of
the Meridians, their pathways, direction, and points.

In this lesson we shall deal with the first and last points of each Meridian; we shall only broadly indicate the path. Later on, each Meridian will be taken in turn, and in thorough detail.

Each Meridian particularly associated with a special inner organ, function, process or system, takes the name of that organ, function, etc. There are twelve of these "Organ Meridians". They are bi-lateral, which is to say, they have symmetrical pathways, one on either side of the body.

Two other pathways, not organ meridians, but which have certain features making it expedient to classify them as Meridians are distinguished from the organ meridians by being named 'Median Vessel Meridians'. These are not bi-lateral, but run up the middle line of the body, one in front and one behind.

We now give the names of the twelve organ meridians, allotting to each a number (in Roman numerals), indicating the direction of flow of vital energy, and the placing of the first and last points. Remember that the energy circulates continuously; and the allotting of numbers to the meridians does not indicate order of importance, neither does it indicate a beginning and end of the circulation — a circulation is continuous — it is simply a matter of expediency where we choose to begin our consideration of the circulatory flow.

The Heart Meridian I   [See page 29]

This meridian begins on the trunk, right up in the apex of the armpit — technically described: 'In the apex of the axilla, below the outer border of the first rib, on the axillary artery where this can be felt pulsating between the subscapularis and coracobrachialis muscles and the tendons of the latissimus dorsi.'

The path then goes down the arm and forearm on the side nearest to the body (i.e. antero-medically) to finish at the root of the little finger nail, ring, finger side. This is the last, the 9th point of the heart meridian (I.9). See chart.

(It is taken for granted that the subject is standing in the "anatomical position" — a position in which no one ever seems to stand naturally, i.e. erect, arms hanging by the sides with the palms of the hands facing forwards!)

The Small Intestine Meridian II   [See pages 51, 56, 58]

This has its first point on the little finger at the root of the fingernail (see chart), it then travels up the postero-internal aspect of the arm, over the shoulder to the face where it has its last, the 19th point (II.19), just anterior to the tragus. See chart.

The Bladder Meridian III   [See pages 105-112]

This has its first point on the face, just medial to the inner corner of the eye (see chart). N.B. It is forbidden to cauterize at this point, i.e. forbidden to Moxa.

The word 'Moxa' is simply the anglicised form of the Japanese mokusu, meaning 'burning herb', and refers to a treatment technique which we shall be dealing with later on in the course.

The path of the bladder meridian goes over the head, down the back of the neck, back, back of thighs and legs to finish at the root of the nail of the little toe (see chart), this last point is the 67th point (III.67).

The Kidneys Meridian IV   [See pages 115-119]

This meridian begins on the sole of the foot, the 1st point being between the pads formed at the base of the big toe and the other toes (see chart). The pathway then goes up the inner aspect of leg and thigh, up the front of the abdomen and thorax to its last point, the 27th (IV.27) just below the clavicle in the triangular hollow formed by the clavicle, first rib, and sternum (see chart).

The Circulation Meridian V   [See pages 37-39]

It begins on the thorax, lateral to the nipple (see chart), goes to the arm, down the anterior of the arm and forearm, over the palm to its last, the 9th, point (V.9) which is at the root of the nail of the middle finger (see chart).

Note: This is the only meridian on which there are no forbidden points.

The Three-Heater Meridian VI   [See pages 51-55]

This meridian begins with its first point at the nail root of the ring finger, little finger side (see chart), goes up the back of the forearm, arm, over the back of the shoulder, round the ear to the last, the 23rd, point (VI.23) which is near the outer extremity of the eyebrow (see chart).

N.B. This point (VI.23) is forbidden to Moxa.

The Gall or Gall Bladder Meridian VII   [See pages 124-131]

Here the Meridian starts with its 1st point just behind the outer corner of the eye, vertically below VI.23 (see chart), the path goes back and forth over the skull, forward over the shoulder, down the side of the thorax and abdomen, down the outer side of the thigh and leg to the last, the 44th, point (VII.44) which is at the root of the fourth toe nail (see chart).

The Liver Meridian VIII   [See pages 135-140]

The liver meridian begins on the big toe at the root of the toenail, 2nd toe side (see chart), goes up the inner surface of leg and thigh, and up the abdomen to finish at its 14th point (VIII.14) on the costal border where this is intersected by a vertical line drawn down from the nipple (see chart).

The Lungs Meridian IX   [See pages 43-45]

The lungs meridian begins in the first intercostal space on the continuation of the paraxillary line (see chart), the path goes down the antero-lateral aspect of the arm to its last point at the root of the thumb nail: this last point, the 11th (IX.11), is forbidden to Moxa (see chart).

The Large Intestine Meridian X   [See pages 45-49]

Beginning at the root of the first fingernail (see chart), the colon meridian goes up the postero-lateral of forearm and arm, over the shoulder, neck and face to finish at the side of the nostril (see chart); this, the 20th point (X.20), is forbidden to Moxa.

The Stomach Meridian XI   [See pages 145-151]

According to Dr. Wu Wei Ping, the stomach meridian has its first point at the centre of the lower edge of the orbital cavity, vertically below the centre of the pupil (see chart). This point is forbidden to Moxa.

(Most European authorities consider the stomach meridian as beginning of the forehead at what Dr. Wu Wei Ping calls its 8th point.)

The meridian goes over the face to the forehead, then down to the throat, the front of the thorax, abdomen, anterior of thigh and leg to finish with the 45th point (XI.45) at the root of the 2nd toe nail (little toe side). See chart.

The Spleen Meridian XII   [See pages 152-157]

The spleen meridian begins at the root of the big toe nail (see chart) (N.B. this 1st point is forbidden to Moxa), the path goes up the internal aspect of the leg and thigh, crosses the groin, up the abdomen and thorax to finish at its 21st point (XII.21) in the 6th intercostal space on the axillary line.

The Vessel Meridians

The two median vessel meridians do not form part of the organ meridian circulation, and we do not, therefore, allot a number to them, but refer to them by their names.

The anterior median vessel meridian is called the 'Conception Vessel'. This has its 1st point in the exact centre of the perineum (this point is forbidden to Moxa). The path follows the anterior median line up the abdomen, sternum, and throat to finish just below the lower lip, its 24th point.

The posterior median vessel meridian is called 'the Governor Vessel'. This has its first point just beyond the tip of the coccyx. The path follows up the centre of the spinous processes, over the middle line of the head, down the middle line of forehead and nose and top lip, to the 28th point which is inside the mouth, on the front of the upper gum between the roots of the two front teeth.

All information in this section must be thoroughly understood; and the location of the points, meridian names, numbers, and general direction must be memorized. These 1st and last points are both diagnostically and therapeutically of great importance. Make sure that you know whether a point is forbidden or not, if it is forbidden, then to what action (needle or moxa).

The First and Last Points of the Meridians

Each of the meridians will be taken in turn in subsequent lessons, and in considerable detail, and it will therefore be sufficient if I give a few notes about some of the first and last points.

According to acupuncture tradition, built up over several thousand years, a symptom occurring on or near the point at one extremity of a meridian may be effectively treated by acting on the point at the other, the opposite extremity. Also, damage to the area at or near one extreme of a meridian will often have repercussions at the opposite extremity of that meridian. This has been confirmed more than once in my own experience.

The first instance I will tell you about represents an almost perfect example of "opposite-ends-reaction". The patient had to be treated by a dentist, to have one of the upper canines drilled and stopped. The last point of the large intestine meridian, X.20, practically coincides with the root tip of this tooth. The patient was instructed to treat herself by finger nail pressure at the 1st point of this meridian, X.1, while she was in the chair. This she did. The tooth was drilled and dealt with, without local anaesthetic, and she did not experience pain while the work was going on.

Two other instances occur to me of the use of this point, X.1, which is sometimes known as "the dentist's point".

In one case, a woman, whose teeth were all in excellent condition, accidentally shut the last phalange of her first finger in a window, damaging the area close to the nail root. Within three weeks, not only did she have toothache (an experience hitherto unknown to her) but signs of a small abscess at the tooth root of one of the upper incisors appeared. The other case was about a child at the "tooth-changing age". One of the second teeth was apparently trying hard to push its way through, but the first tooth just would not loosen and give way. The child accidentally shut one of his forefingers in the door "dead on" the 1st point of the large intestine meridian. That same day the obstinate tooth loosened and fell out. By accident the lad had treated himself in accordance with the best acupuncture tradition.

Pains, inflammations, sores, and so on very close to the eyes make local treatment by acupuncture impossible and inadvisable. In these instances one treats the point at the opposite end of the Meridian most closely concerned, e.g. III.67, XI.45, VII.44, or VI.1.

One patient complained of such a dry mouth that she found it difficult to chew and swallow — there was not enough saliva. She was also troubled with itching around the outer corner of the eyelids. This is close to the 1st point of the gall meridian. The 44th, the last point, of this meridian was selected for treatment. As she walked out of the room she held her handkerchief to her mouth laughingly saying, ''That has most certainly done the trick — I cannot stop my mouth watering now!''

It is an inflexible rule that local action must not be taken on a tumour or swelling. Thus, if a tumour, boil, abscess, inflammation of a serious nature, etc., occurs on or very close to one end of a meridian, the point of selection for treatment could be at the opposite end of that meridian.

The finger and toe nail points have many, many other uses, some of these being given as this course proceeds.

FIRST POINTS ON THE THORAX

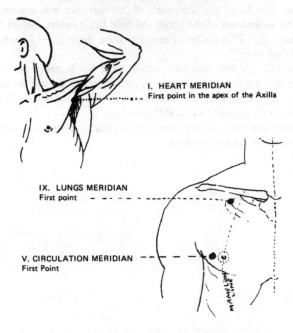

I. HEART MERIDIAN
First point in the apex of the Axilla

IX. LUNGS MERIDIAN
First point

V. CIRCULATION MERIDIAN
First Point

MAMELON LINE

LAST POINTS ON THE THORAX

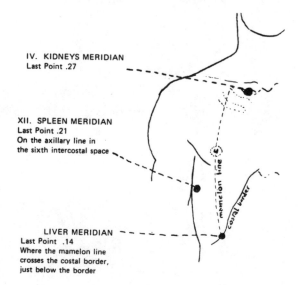

IV. KIDNEYS MERIDIAN
Last Point .27

XII. SPLEEN MERIDIAN
Last Point .21
On the axillary line in
the sixth intercostal space

mamelon line

costal border

LIVER MERIDIAN
Last Point .14
Where the mamelon line
crosses the costal border,
just below the border

NOTE: All points are bi-lateral, but only one side is shown.

FIRST AND LAST POINTS ON THE FEET

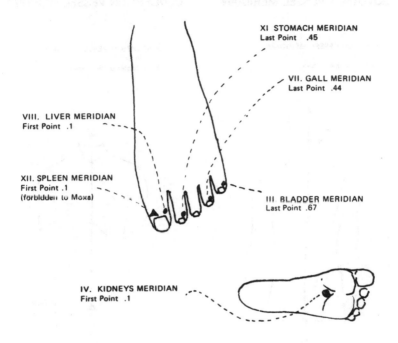

XI STOMACH MERIDIAN
Last Point .45

VII. GALL MERIDIAN
Last Point .44

VIII. LIVER MERIDIAN
First Point .1

XII. SPLEEN MERIDIAN
First Point .1
(forbidden to Moxa)

III BLADDER MERIDIAN
Last Point .67

IV. KIDNEYS MERIDIAN
First Point .1

FIRST AND LAST POINTS ON THE HAND

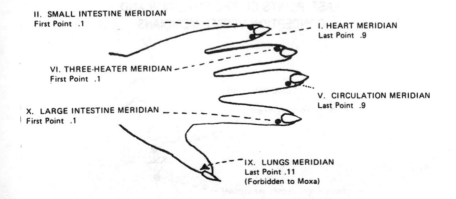

II. SMALL INTESTINE MERIDIAN
First Point .1

I. HEART MERIDIAN
Last Point .9

VI. THREE-HEATER MERIDIAN
First Point .1

V. CIRCULATION MERIDIAN
Last Point .9

X. LARGE INTESTINE MERIDIAN
First Point .1

IX. LUNGS MERIDIAN
Last Point .11
(Forbidden to Moxa)

FIRST POINT OF THE GOVERNOR VESSEL MERIDIAN

FIRST POINT OF THE CONCEPTION VESSEL MERIDIAN

GOVERNOR VESSEL MERIDIAN
First Point .1
At the tip of the coccyx

CONCEPTION VESSEL MERIDIAN
First Point .1
In the center of the perineum

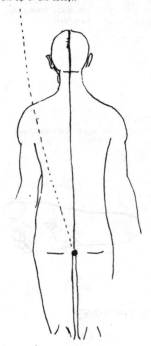

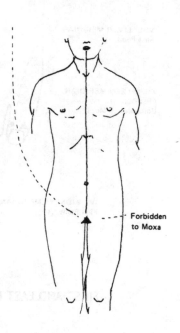

- - - Forbidden to Moxa

LAST POINTS OF THE GOVERNOR AND CONCEPTION VESSEL MERIDIANS

GOVERNOR VESSEL MERIDIAN
Last point .28
Inside the mouth on the gum

CONCEPTION VESSEL MERIDIAN
Last Point .24

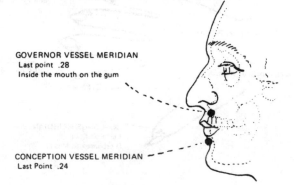

FIRST POINTS ON THE FACE

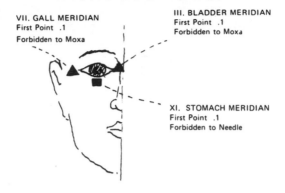

VII. GALL MERIDIAN
First Point .1
Forbidden to Moxa

III. BLADDER MERIDIAN
First Point .1
Forbidden to Moxa

XI. STOMACH MERIDIAN
First Point .1
Forbidden to Needle

LAST POINTS ON THE FACE

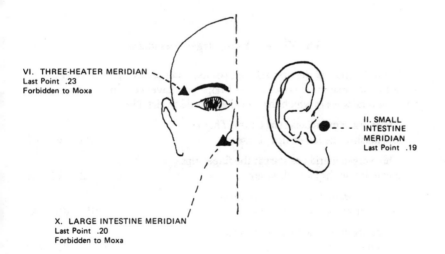

VI. THREE-HEATER MERIDIAN
Last Point .23
Forbidden to Moxa

II. SMALL
INTESTINE
MERIDIAN
Last Point .19

X. LARGE INTESTINE MERIDIAN
Last Point .20
Forbidden to Moxa

2

The Yin and Yang Organ Meridians

From the chart of the first and last points, and the descriptions, brief though they were, you may have noticed (and I hope you have) certain groupings which offer us several ways in which the meridians could be classified.

Three organ meridians start on the Thorax
and finish at the finger-tips: these are   I.   V.   IX.

Three organ meridians start at the finger-tips
and finish on the face: these are   II.   VI.   X.

Three organ meridians start on the face
and finish at the toes: these are   III.   VII.   XI.

Three organ meridians start at the feet
and finish on the thorax: these are   IV.   VIII.   XII.

This can be further simplified by considering, as regards general direction of flow, that six meridians have the flow going outwards towards the extremities, namely:

I.   III.   V.   VII.   IX.   XI.

the direction of flow in these is centrifugal.

Six of the meridians have the flow going inwards from the extremities towards the body; namely:

II. IV. VI. VIII. X. XII.

the direction of flow in these is centripetal.

Just as a memory aid — Odd numbers centrifugal,
Even numbers centripetal.

Each centrifugal organ meridian is intimately linked with the centripetal organ meridian following it. Thus, we have an important pairing of the organ meridians:

I & II, III & IV, V & VI, VII & VIII, IX & X, XI & XII.

There is a characteristic of these pairs that you will not have been able to deduce from what has so far been given you in the first lesson. This we shall now go into:

Each organ meridian is classified as a Yin or a Yang organ meridian; and in each pair one is Yin and the other is Yang. This needs some explanation.

It means that the polarity of the energy is predominantly one or the other polarity. The energy is only one energy, and always has both polarities, but one of these polarities predominates.

If we now write the list of the Yin organ meridians, and a list of the Yang organ meridians, and compare them, we shall be able to see an important difference between them.

The Yin organ meridians are these:
I heart; IV kidneys; V circulation; VIII liver; IX lungs; and XII spleen.

The Yang organ meridians are these:
II small intestine; III bladder; VI three-heater; VII gall bladder; X large intestine; and XI stomach.

The important difference that we observe from this classification is that all the Yang organs are concerned with nutrition (food) & excretion or alimentation and elimination. These are concerned with the conversion of environment, taken in as food and drink, into an energy form assimilable by the organism; or to cast out into the environment waste products and any unassimilable matter. De la Fuye calls these the workshop or manufactory organs.

All the Yin organs are concerned with the storage and distribution or circulation of the assimilated energy. These de la Fuye calls the treasury organs.

In the Nei Ching, the Yellow Emperor's Classic of Internal Medicine (several thousand years old) we are told that is the function of Yin to preserve Yang; which means that the Yin organs store the energy supplied through the Yang organs.

The time has come to put this in tabular form:

PAIRS OF MERIDIANS	PREDOMINANT POLARITY	DIRECTION OF FLOW	LIMBS
I	Yin	Centrifugal	Arms
II	Yang	Centripetal	
III	Yang	Centrifugal	Legs
IV	Yin	Centripetal	
V	Yin	Centrifugal	Arms
VI	Yang	Centripetal	
VII	Yang	Centrifugal	Legs
VIII	Yin	Centripetal	
IX	Yin	Centrifugal	Arms
X	Yang	Centripetal	
XI	Yang	Centrifugal	Legs
XII	Yin	Centripetal	

Note and remember that the energy changes its polarity characteristic on passing from a meridian to the meridian with which it is paired, and this change occurs at the limb extremities.

The energy does not change its polarity characteristic when it passes from the last of one pair to the first of the next pair. This passing from one pair to the next occurs on the trunk or face.

Try to get a clear picture of this, and tuck it away safely at the back of your mind, so that when we come to the five elements law you will have it already well and truly established in your memory.

We could have arranged our acupuncture anatomy study by simply taking one meridian after another in numerical order, detailing the points; or we could have arranged it so that we took one pair at a time. There are many ways in which it could have been presented to you. But I have given the matter   careful thought, and tried to arrange the sequence of presentation in such a way as to simplify the study for you as much as possible, especially in these early lessons.

We shall start our detailed acupuncture anatomy study of the meridians and their points with an examination of the shortest organ meridians, followed by the detailed study of the three organ meridians paired with them. After that we shall be taking the remaining meridians in numerical order, thereby completing a pair with each two meridians taken.

The conception and governor vessel meridians will be taken together at an appropriate time.

This is not the usual procedure when teaching acupuncture, but from teaching experience I have come to the conclusion that the more conventional way is also the dry-as-dust way. It is the aim of this book to make the study as interesting as we can, and in so doing automatically make learning easier.

The Heart Meridian (I)
And the   Acupuncture   Unit of Measurement (A.U.M.)

Our detailed study of points begins with the shortest of all organ meridians — the heart meridian (I), which begins on the thorax and goes down the arm to the hand. It has nine points.

In his Treatise on Acupuncture, the late Dr. Roger de la Fuye underlined the importance of this organ meridian by pointing out that the greatest objection put forward by western anatomists to the existence of the meridians and the direction of energy current in them is that the meridians do not follow any anatomical path known to western anatomy: nerve, artery, or vein. But he says it is common knowledge that angina pectoris pain follows a path from the heart to little finger, even though there is no anatomically explicable link between the heart and the little finger — and this path coincides exactly with the traditional path of the heart meridian. The reality of the heart meridian may not be demonstrable by dissection, but it can be proved on a living person.

But wait a minute — before we get in a mess!

How are we going to set about describing the exact position of acupuncture points? What standard of measurement can be used that will be valid for a child or an adult, for a dwarf or a giant?

Thousands of years ago, the Chinese solved this difficulty of accurate description without having to go into highly complex and minute anatomical details of the 'under the skin' structures. They devised a flexible unit, a 'Chinese inch', which varies from person to person, and from one part of the body to another and yet is always valid.

In this course we refer to the standard unit of measurement as: the acupuncture unit of measurement, which we abbreviate by using the initial letters A.U.M.

For any given individual this A.U.M. will be constant, although even on the individual allowance has to be made for his personal variations. There is, therefore, a standard technique for doing this. Once you have mastered it, and it is extremely easy to master, you will be able to pinpoint the acupuncture points with quite extraordinary precision.

THE ACUPUNCTURE UNIT OF MEASUREMENT

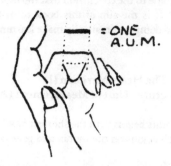

= ONE
A.U.M.

Some of the French schools and German schools of acupuncture take as the standard the width of the last phalange of the middle finger of the patient, the finger being pressed firmly on a flat surface. In an average adult this is about 2 centimetres; thus, one sometimes comes across the measurements quoted in centimetres.

Far Eastern tradition, however, does not take the finger width as the standard; but takes the distance between the ends of the outer folds (thumb side) formed at the articulations of the first and second, and the second and third phalanges of the fully flexed middle finger. (See diagram.) Take this measurement on the left hand for a male, and on the right for a female, and that represents the standard A.U.M. for that person. Even this A.U.M. has some variations which have to be taken into account; for there will be a variation applicable to special parts of the body or limbs. In order to ascertain these special applications certain clearly defined reference points are taken, the distance between them is measured and divided into a number of equal divisions. We shall not list all these now, but only take them as they are needed in our actual study.

On the upper limb the reference points are these:

The anterior fold of the axilla, upper extremity, where this vertical line meets the horizontal line made by the lower border of the pectoralis major (see diagram).

The Deltoid 'V', which is the place where the deltoid tendon attaches to the humerus, between the triceps lateral head and the biceps.

The Elbow fold, usually the outer extremity is taken when measuring to the deltoid 'V', and the inner extremity when measuring to the axilla fold (anterior).

The Wrist fold, this being marked by the crease formed on flexing the wrist.

On the heart meridian it will be more convenient to use the deltoid 'V' reference point, so our next step is for you to mark this. Wind (or wrap) a suitable length of tape round the arm at the level of the deltoid 'V'; with a dermographic pencil draw a line right round the arm.

Now flex the elbow fully and make a mark at either extremity of the elbow crease. Extend the arm at the elbow, and draw a line joining the two marks you have just made, following the actual crease line.

I. HEART MERIDIAN

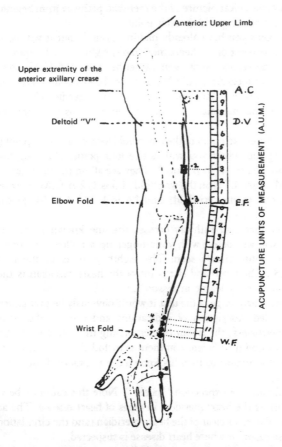

Anterior: Upper Limb

Upper extremity of the
anterior axillary crease

Deltoid "V"

Elbow Fold

Wrist Fold

A.C

D.V

E.F.

W.F.

ACUPUNCTURE UNITS OF MEASUREMENT (A.U.M.)

The distance between the deltoid 'V' line and the elbow fold line is divided into seven equal parts, each division counting as one A.U.M.

From the elbow fold to the wrist fold is taken as measuring twelve A.U.M.

When describing the location of acupuncture points, the points are said to be a certain number of A.U.M. from one reference point to another.

Referring to your chart, mark in dermographic pencil the path of the heart meridian from one end to the other. From the apex of the axilla the path goes vertically down the inner surface of the arm, practically following the straight line of the intermuscular septum to the inner extremity of the elbow fold. From here the path goes down the antero-internal aspect to the wrist fold where the ulnar artery can be felt pulsating. This will be just proximal to the pisiform. From here the path goes over the hypothenar eminence towards the base of the little finger, ring finger side, and thence gradually curving round the little finger to finish at the external ungueal angle of the little finger (ring finger side). (See chart.)

You now have a clear picture of the meridian pathway from beginning to end, and you can set about marking each point.

The first point you have already had in Lesson I, but it will do no harm to repeat it; the first point of the heart meridian is right up in the apex of the axilla.

To locate the second point, you can either take 4 A.U.M. down from the deltoid 'V' line, or measure 3 A.U.M. up from the elbow fold. Here is I.2. *Never use a needle at this point.* This point is forbidden to needle. This is the only forbidden point on this meridian. The heart meridian has no points forbidden to moxa.

The exact inner extremity of the elbow fold locates the third point (I.3).

Consulting your chart you will notice four points close together near the wrist. These are points, 4, 5, 6, and 7. They are all on the ulnar artery; they are half an A.U.M. apart. I.7 is on the wristfold; I.6 is 1/2 A.U.M. proximal; I.5 is 1 A.U.M. proximal to the wristfold; and I.4 is 1 1/2 A.U.M. proximal to the wristfold.

Where the meridian pathway crosses the line known in palmistry as the "heart line" you will detect with your finger tip a hollow; in some people the hollow may be quite clearly seen. The eighth point is in the centre of this depression (I.8). The ninth and last point of the heart meridian is the fingernail point you have already learnt in lesson I.

At this very early stage of the text it would obviously be premature to embark upon any detailed description of indications and uses of the points on this meridian. Nevertheless, the labour of memorising the meridians and their points is considerably eased if sufficient comment is included to sustain a varied interest and to enable the student to turn his knowledge to practical use as early as may safely be done.

I do emphasize the expression "safely". Note this caution: be very careful indeed about using the heart meridian in cases of heart disease. The acupuncture novice is advised to steer clear of the heart meridian (and the circulation meridian) in heart disease cases, or where heart disease is suspected.

According to the wise masters of acupuncture there is only one safe way to treat heart disease by acupuncture; and that is by what is known as 'applying the five elements laws'.

All the same, this meridian, the heart meridian, is of especial value for the treatment of certain psychological and/or emotional states. One can treat nervous anxiety and the symptoms that go with this state after further studies.

As an example: I.5 and I.7 are especially useful for the nervous anxiety known as 'stage fright' or 'examination nerves'. This anxiety tends to be characterised by palpitations, and even goes so far as to produce a sudden inability to speak. When this sudden inability to speak results from an emotional shock, the three points I.4, I.5, I.6 may all be massaged together, and including I.7 with good effect.

I.7 used by itself is suitable in cases of sleeplessness due to mental over-activity, nervous restlessness and anxiety.

When there is the kind of headache that goes with loss of appetite, and all joy seems to have gone out of life, the third point, I.3, would be the point of selection on this meridian. In my own experience, I have known one treatment at this point (I.3) to have lifted almost at once a deep depression and feeling of utter hopelessness, and to my knowledge this depressed, joyless gloom has not returned, and three years have gone by since the treatment was given. Dr. de la Fuye nicknamed this point ''joi de vivre'', and it certainly seems to merit this nickname.

If mental tone is low, and there is a corresponding feeling of depression, reduced intellectual acuity, and consequent lack of interest, inability to focus attention and so on, the tone can be considerably raised by treating just this single point, I.9, the last point of the heart meridian.

In addition to a wide range of emotional and psychological disturbances where one of the principal features is repercussion on the heart itself, e.g. palpitation, arhythmy, etc., there is also a number of local conditions where the heart meridian would be used.

Although we shall be going into this more fully later on in the course, it is as well for you to realize that some symptoms, especially skin or muscular, are often very effectively treated at points quite close to the actual site of the symptom. As, for example, arthritic pain in the elbow is treatable at I.4; this would be when the pain and inflammation is centered around the 3rd point of the heart meridian. Energy excess and congestion which causes the pain is drained away from the painful area by acting upon the nearest point distal to the elbow, namely I.4.

There is an important general principle to be memorized, namely: according to Far-Oriental tradition and medicine-philosophy, *all palliatives or symptom-suppressive treatments are, in principle, to be avoided and if, in cases of emergency or expediency, a palliative is used, it should be used only in order to facilitate treatment of deep or root cause of the disturbance.*

The Far-Eastern practitioner aims to remove root causes and not merely to suppress symptoms. In the West, however, a great deal of symptomatic treatment will be called for; therefore, never lose sight of the guiding principle.

In the next lesson we shall begin to study the characteristic diagnostic technique of acupuncture, namely the pulses technique.

3

The 12 Pulses

By the time you come to read this Lesson you should have some understanding of the Energy concepts — the notions of the One Energy with its two polarities, Yin and Yang. If, as we have said, the individual is in health so long as there is a proper or normal balance, and the various rhythms, and changes are happening at their proper time — and ill health results from a disturbed balance — then it is obviously of paramount importance to us to be able to assess whether, in our patient, the balance is as it should be. How.is this to be done?

Thousands of years before the Christian Era the Chinese recognized that there was a definite relationship between the heartbeat, respiration rhythm, and blood flow. This relationship reflected the state of health of the organism as a whole. This is also acknowledged in Western Medicine; and it is an essential part of any clinical examination to note breathing — how many breaths to the minute, is the breathing shallow or deep, even or irregular? — the heartbeat — how many beats to each breath, strong or weak, even or irregular? — and the blood flow, when it is felt where a blood vessel is conveniently near the surface, is the flow full or thin, strong or weak, hard or soft, regular or intermittent, etc?

To most Westerners, when one mentions "taking a patient's pulse" attention at once goes to the wrist, where the radial artery can easily be felt pulsating. There are several other places where the pulsations can be just as easily felt; in fact, wherever an artery runs close to a bone and near to the skin, thus being easily compressible.

The truly great discovery made by the Chinese, as regards the pulse, was that *through the pulse it is possible to read not merely the health of the organism as a whole, but that of each inner organ separately* — whether it had much or little energy, whether it was congested, over-full, or escaping, deficient; whether it was hyper or hypo active; whether the polarity predominance and polarity changes were in proper order, and so on.

They discovered, quite early in their medicine-history, that at the wrist twelve different pulse phenomena were discernible — six upon each wrist, upon the radial artery.

There are, according to Tradition, three positions upon each wrist; and at each position two levels or depths (a superficial and a deep). At each level, at each position on either wrist a different inner state is reflected.

Before I go on to describe the exact location of each of the twelve Pulses recognized in Acupuncture, and the organs associated with them, let us first see whether the notions of two levels and three positions can make any sort of sense to us.

It is important that you should test for yourself the fact of differences, and appreciate the logic of it all.

I do urge you not to let it rest at just reading the words of these paragraphs — words by themselves may be quite unconvincing — but practical experience will serve to confirm the reality of differences in a way that no words of mine (nor of anyone else) can.

If we have a fluid flowing through a resilient tube, a rubber or plastic tube attached to a water tap, and very lightly touch the tube with a finger, the flow of water can be felt. The tube need hardly be compressed at all for us to feel the flow quite distinctly. Let the finger tip linger awhile, so that the kind of sensation of flow registers in you; now steadily compress the tube by increasing the pressure until you have almost stopped the flow, then lift ever so slightly — maintain this pressure and note: the kind of sensation you now experience in your finger tip is different from that of the first light touch. You may, for example, be more aware of the resilience of the tube itself, at one pressure level rather than another; or of volume, water pressure, speed of flow, etc.

Continue your experiment by varying the surface upon which the tube rests. A tube resting upon a hard surface will feel different from when it is resting upon a soft surface. This will apply to both levels.

How soon you will be able to detect a flow will vary according to what layers of material there might be between your finger tip and the tube. You will soon realize that it is far from nonsensical to suggest that a pulse felt superficially in one place can give a noticeably different reading from a pulse position only a finger's width away, higher up or lower down the same artery.

Turn to the diagrams and have a good look at the relevant drawings.

In the West one is so accustomed to have everything tested and proved by meter readings of one kind or another, that it would not surprise me if you wondered whether the pulse differences are recordable on a meter. I have actually tested this for myself over and over again on patients, using the ordinary clinical sphygmomanometer. In order to play absolutely fair in making my tests, the meter scale was faced away from me, so that I could not read the meter myself — I simply told my assistant the moment to read off from the scale.

With a sphygmomanometer one gets only a relatively crude and limited recorded difference — not the fine qualitative differences detectable through one's fingers — but even if 'sphyg' readings are not usable in acupuncture, at least it gives instrumental confirmation of the fact of differences.

Using the 'sphyg' I have had twelve different readings at the same session, the lowest 85, the highest 160, the others ranging at uneven intervals between. Instrumentally, one may well get several of the readings similar, just as with the fingers one may assess several pulses as normal.

In acupuncture we do not use instruments for pulse reading — we use our finger tips.

The chart illustrates the traditional pulse positions, depths, and organs to which they correspond. These must be learned and known so thoroughly that there is never, never any doubt in your mind as to what organ pulse you are feeling.

First, learn to read your own pulses. You will have to do this so many times in the course of your practice, because, according to Tradition, the practitioner uses his own pulses as the standard by which he assesses those of his patient. No wonder the Far East tradition demands the healer to be a model of good health himself, and to set an example to his patient. A practitioner in poor health should not give Acupuncture treatment, let alone diagnose.

Sit relaxed. With your right hand feel the pulses of your left hand. In order to do this, rest the back of the left wrist on the palm of the right hand and curl the fingers over so as to rest upon the radial artery. See illustration. Place the middle finger at the level of the bony prominence just below the wrist fold; the forefinger will then rest naturally on the fold, itself, close to the thenar eminence; the ring finger again will fall naturally into the correct third position.

On the Left Hand

Position 1	*is the position nearest to the thumb and is felt with the forefinger.*
Position 2	*is felt with the middle finger.*
Position 3	*is felt with the ring finger.*

Light pressure at Position 1 detects the superficial pulse, which is the Pulse of the Small Intestine (II). Deep pressure reveals the deep pulse, which is that of the heart.

Light pressure at Position 2 detects the superficial pulse, which is the Pulse of the Gall Bladder (VIII), while deep pressure reveals the dep pulse which is that of the Liver (VIII).

Light pressure at Position 3 detects the superficial pulse, which is the pulse of the Bladder (III), while deep pressure reveals the Pulse of the Kidneys (IV).

This should be easy enough to remember: First Finger — First Position. The superficial pulses are those of YANG organs, while the deep pulses are those of YIN organs.

THE TWELVE RADIAL PULSES OF CHINESE ACUPUNCTURE

LEFT HAND

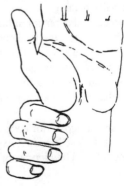

$\left.\begin{array}{l}1^{st} \\ 2^{nd} \\ 3^{rd}\end{array}\right\}$ position ① ② ③

1. $\left\{\begin{array}{l}\text{Superficial}\\\text{SMALL INTESTINE, II.}\\\text{Deep}\\\text{HEART,} \qquad \text{I.}\end{array}\right.$

2. $\left\{\begin{array}{l}\text{Superficial}\\\text{GALL BLADDER, VII.}\\\text{Deep}\\\text{LIVER,} \qquad \text{VIII}\end{array}\right.$

3. $\left\{\begin{array}{l}\text{Superficial}\\\text{BLADDER,} \quad \text{III.}\\\text{Deep}\\\text{KIDNEYS,} \quad \text{IV.}\end{array}\right.$

HOW TO FEEL YOUR OWN PULSES

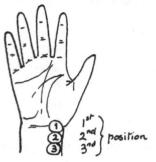

THE TWELVE RADIAL PULSES OF CHINESE ACUPUNCTURE

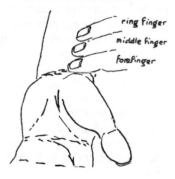

① ② ③ $\left.\begin{array}{l}1^{st} \\ 2^{nd} \\ 3^{rd}\end{array}\right\}$ position

1. $\left.\begin{array}{l}\text{Superficial}\\\text{LARGE INTESTINE, X.}\\\text{Deep}\\\text{LUNGS,} \qquad \text{IX}\end{array}\right\}$

2. $\left.\begin{array}{l}\text{Superficial}\\\text{STOMACH, XI}\\\text{Deep}\\\text{SPLEEN, XII}\end{array}\right\}$

3. $\left.\begin{array}{l}\text{Superficial}\\\text{THREE-HEATER, VI.}\\\text{Deep}\\\text{CIRCULATION, V.}\end{array}\right\}$

HOW TO FEEL A PATIENT'S PULSES

ring finger
middle finger
forefinger

The same will apply when you change hands to feel the pulses of the right hand.

On the Right Hand

Position 1	superficial	Large Intestine
	deep	lungs
Position 2	superficial	Stomach
	deep	Spleen
Position 3	superficial	Three Heater
	deep	Circulation

Let us repeat: ALL superficial pulses relate to YANG, and deep pulses to YIN organs.

Feel your own pulses: feel them over and over again, each day, several times a day, until you are able to detect differences.

Do not, at this stage, try to interpret any differences you may feel. It will suffice that you are able to detect differences.

Some people seem to have a natural ability for this, and can notice differences the very first time — others take a little longer. Generally speaking, only a little practice suffices to detect differences; but it takes a long time and a great deal of practice to become proficient at reading and interpreting with a high degree of skill and artistry.

A word of consolation here: when you are taking your own pulses do not feel anxious or disturbed if one or more of the twelve pulses is scarcely discernible, or if one is much stronger than you expected it to be. This does NOT necessarily mean a disturbance — it may even indicate that that particular pulse, at that hour of the day, at that season of the year, and in relation to other circumstances, is just what it should be.

Get into the habit of glancing at your watch, and the calendar, whenever you feel a pulse. We shall be going into the reasons for this later on. On a patient's Case Sheet always enter the time and date with the pulse reading.

When you have begun to make headway in detecting differences in fulness or emptyness, strength or weakness, hardness or softness, etc., try to describe the differences you feel. Remember, no one is at your elbow to tell you whether you are "right" or "wrong"; there is no one to prompt you into imagining you are feeling what you think they expect you to feel. All you are asked to do is to be receptive to detect what is, in fact, happening — what this is does not matter — simply try to describe what you feel.

Test yourself and write down one of three simple scores for each of your own pulses; that is to say: Normal, Above Normal, Below Normal; expressed by the single letters N = Normal, E = Excess, D = Deficiency, or Below Normal.

The Circulation Meridian [V]

The next Organ Meridian we shall consider in detail is called the Circulation meridian (V). This is a Yin organ meridian. You remember the Yin organs function continuously, and are concerned with storage and distribution. Western physiology does not recognize this as an inner organ. The Far East doctors do. They consider the whole vascular system (arteries, veins, and all vessels dealing with the circulation of fluids throughout the system) to be sufficiently distinct as to merit classification as an organ. It is not located neatly and compactly in one place, as might be the liver or stomach — but the fact of being spread over a large area is no valid argument against its being an organ. Its function is to store and distribute blood and blood-energy (blood, whether oxygenated, deoxygenated, chylifemous, or otherwise).

The First Point on Meridian V has been described in the First Lesson. Nevertheless, now that we have learned (in Lesson 2) about the A.U.M., we can describe the location of V.1 a little differently. V.1 is 1 A.U.M. lateral to the mamelon; or, as some authorities describe it, 1 finger's width lateral to the edge of the mamelon areola, in the fourth intercostal space.

The path ascends and curves outwards around the anterior axillary fold and, closely parallel to the Heart meridian, follows vertically downwards along the upper internal tendon of the brachial biceps, down the antero-internal of the biceps to the internal side of the tendon of insertion of this muscle, where the path then crosses the elbow fold.

The second point of the Circulation meridian is on the upper arm exactly at the horizontal level of the Deltoid V. This reference point you will have located and used in Lesson 2.

The third point, V.3, is on the elbow fold itself in the small hollow internal to the biceps tendon of insertion. See Chart.

From the Elbow Fold the path follows the interstice between the flexor carpi radialis and palmaris longus to about half way to the wrist; it then follows alongside the tendon of the flexor sublimis digitorum to the wrist fold.

As you recall, E.F. to W.F. = 12 A.U.M.
The seventh point, V.7, is at the middle of the W.F.
5 A.U.M above the W.F.is the fourth point, V.4.
3 A.U.M. above the W.F. is the fifth point, V.5.
2 A.U.M. above the W.F. is the sixth point, V.6.

From the seventh point on the wrist fold the path goes over the palm to the centre, V.8, then curving obliquely goes towards, and then the length of, the external (thumbside) border of the middle finger to the root of the finger nail, the external ungueal angle, which is its ninth point, V.9. See Chart.

No points at all on this meridian are forbidden. This is not only one of the meridians which may be allowed to bleed, but there is actually a point at which treatment is given to make it bleed, namely at V.3, which is made to bleed in cases of vomiting and diarrhoea.

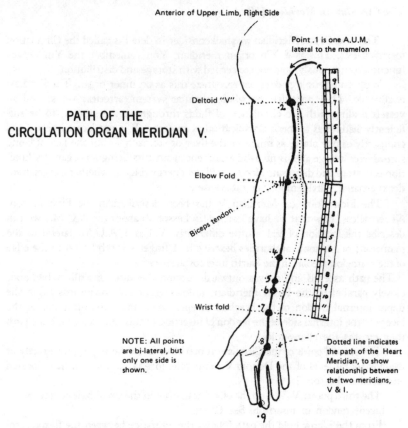

Anterior of Upper Limb, Right Side

Point .1 is one A.U.M. lateral to the mamelon

Deltoid "V"

PATH OF THE CIRCULATION ORGAN MERIDIAN V.

Elbow Fold

Biceps tendon

Wrist fold

NOTE: All points are bi-lateral, but only one side is shown.

Dotted line indicates the path of the Heart Meridian, to show relationship between the two meridians, V & I.

Provided your patient is not too well upholstered, and the muscle and tendon contours are visible, the pathway of this meridian is easily traceable, just by looking at it.

V.6 is one of the Great Points of Acupuncture.

There are, however, only nine points in all on this meridian, so it will not be imposing too great a burden or strain for you to memorize the location and number of each.

Although I have said that V.6 is one of the Great Points, you will not see it figuring prominently in any repertory: but you will find it re-appearing over and over again in the well-tried and tested formulae or special combinations of points which, over the centuries, have been found remarkably effective in special conditions or syndromes. These special formulae will be of immense value to you clinically, so when one is mentioned memorise it. At the moment, we have not yet been through enough of the meridians to warrant any formulae. Point Number V.6 is also one of the Command Points we shall learn when we come to the Five Elements Law method.

There are several uses of V.6, suitable for psychological and/or emotional disturbances; or symptoms arising out of emotional shock. As you know, the menses are often disturbed by shock, as well as by cold baths, etc. V.6 is one of the very effective points to treat disturbed menses, e.g. too early, too long, too copious, arrested, painful, etc. — accidental amenorrhoea such as occurs after shock.

In general, one can say that the ancient Chinese considered that disorders of the sex function have always psychological roots, and therefore this meridian should not be considered in cases of sexual disorders, male and female, but NOT because this meridian is especially linked with the sex-function (as some Western acupuncturists teach) but because it has a powerful effect upon the psyche.

V.7 is a useful point to remember in all skin diseases, whether the skin is inside or outside the body, especially where the symptoms are accompanied by the pulse of this meridian showing an excess or hyperactivity.

One would also use this as the meridian of choice when the vascular tissue is affected, for example, if the artery walls have lost resilience and have hardened. Here the point of selection would be V.8. At this point the vascular tissues, and circulatory system as a whole, can be stimulated, awakened out of lethargy, and, in general, renewed in elasticity and flexibility.

V.5 is a useful point for children who have nightmares. The two meridians detailed so far (Heart, I, and Circulation, V) have peculiar affinity with the speech organs and speech sense, or communication sense. You will readily appreciate how the link with Night Terrors occurs. At the age when a child's speech is coming through, the child begins to dream. It is some time before the child is able to differentiate its dream world from the real world outside. In the early years an incredible amount of psychological adjustments, adaptations, and sorting out takes place — we who are adult seem to lose touch with the tremendous happenings in a child's psyche. The child's Night terrors occur, in effect, because, upon waking from a terrifying dream, the child does not recognize the dream as a dream — and the dream-reality seems to continue on, as if it were a part of the waking state reality.

The congestion, in the psyche, is one of undispersed and undifferentiated excess which seems to need relief from pressure, quietening down, and dispersing to arrive at a proper balance. Ideas, realizations, etc., must circulate freely for them to be adequately sorted out. If this circulation in the Psyche of a young child is congested with an excess that cannot escape, the point, V.5, may be used to assist the maturing process in the psyche. V.5 also is useful for neurasthenia in adults.

In adults, insomnia, due not only to excess activity of blood circulation (which should ease up during sleep), but also to an excess of mental activity or "ideas going round and round in one's head", may be treated at V.7 — this disperses the over-activity and thus promotes relaxation and sleep. When insomnia of this kind occurs the pulse is likely to indicate an excess on the Circulation, V, and at the same time a deficiency on the Lungs, IX, pulses.

4

Reading the Pulse

Having made your first assessments of the twelve pulses and having arrived at the stage when you now notice differences, it is well to indicate how you should set about recording your findings, preparatory to considering what action you should take, if any.

The Chinese allotted a number, a sort of score, to each of the pulse readings. They took "4" as the number of a normal pulse. On the YIN side, the deficient side, the score ranged from 3 to 0. A score of 0 indicated a very serious deficiency; the pulse beat perhaps being almost imperceptible, extremely weak, short, thin, small: could be slow or rapid. Assuming the patient was still alive, it meant that the deficiency was such as to demand action of some sort. A score of 3 would indicate a deficiency, but not necessarily serious, probably enough to be accompanied by symptoms of some sort, though again the only symptom might be the pulse itself. A score of 2 would indicate a state somewhere between 3 and 0.

On the Yang side the figures were taken as 5 to 8. Extreme excess or hyperactivity was represented by the 8. 5 would be used to designate a relatively slight excess, enough to be out of balance, but not necessarily requiring urgent attention as would a pulse assessed at 7.

When feeling pulses the practitioner 'listens' to them much as one might listen to an orchestra — each pulse representing one of the instrumentalists. Taken all together the melody should be harmonious, and a happy one. It is as if you are listening to that person's "life-song". If the melody is not a joyous and harmonious one, and a 'player' is out of tune, the practitioner needs to spot which one is playing out of tune, who is the discordant one, etc.

Pulse assessment is not a matter to be approached roughly and without sensitivity. A highly important rule to be observed is "Silence While Reading The Pulse."

The patient should be relaxed, and have rested for at least ten minutes — preferably longer — to allow plenty of time for the calming down of any emotional excitement, or physical exertion, which would otherwise tend to give misleading pulse readings.

The Chinese considered the ideal time for taking the pulse readings was between 5 a.m. and 1 p.m. But, for obvious reasons, this is not workable always, especially with a busy practice. The various factors to be taken into consideration when reading a pulse include the time of the reading. This I shall go into later on.

The patient should be comfortably reclining, and NOT hopping from one foot to the other. A Master might be able to arrive at a pulse assessment within a few minutes, with the patient standing up and chatting away — but, more often than not, if you see a pulse being taken in this way you can safely bet the practitioner is no Master, and whatever readings he might get would represent a highly unreliable set of information items.

The Practitioner himself must be relaxed, calm and receptive. When he palpates at each position, at each level, he quite deliberately, silently, says to himself, ''I am now listening to the pulse of the Small Intestine (for example), to hear and to try and understand what it is saying to me.''

This almost ritual approach to the reading of pulses has often been sneered at by Westerners who understand so little of Far East wisdom. It does not matter if it takes a whole hour to feel and to assess the pulses. It does not matter if in that hour the pulses are read and re-read several times. It is important to cultivate the ability to listen to the vital message which will become clearly revealed to the calm and RECEPTIVE mind. If this hour is followed by thirty seconds worth of treatment at the right place, more good will have been done for the patient than thirty seconds of diagnosis followed by an hour of treatment!

What is the Life Force doing in each one of the Organs and Organ Meridians? Is there so little Vital Energy that it speaks in the pulse as if it were a thin drawn thread? Is the Energy hurriedly pouring itself away and, as it were, ''the sands rapidly running out''? Is there, somewhere, a blockage against which the Life Force is striving to push its way? Is the ''Life-Effort'' erratic? And so on, and so on?

The human being will tell you, through the pulses, the inmost secrets of the Life Force animating it — and its message will be a truthful message. If the practitioner is sincere and genuinely seeks to understand and receive the message, it will be there. Life always speaks the truth about itself, one simply needs to learn at what level to listen. We shall have more about the pulses later on in the Course. For the present, you will need to practise 'listening' with an open mind, and with an eager sympathetic heart.

The differences you are able to feel today will not be the same as the wide range of subtleties you may be reading in a year or two's time. Accept what you read — whether your reasoning tells you it ought to be different or not. It is not up to the practitioner to dictate to the pulses what message they 'ought' to be giving, and therefore only listen to what he thinks the message should be. The practitioner's task is to read the message as the Life Force in the patient gives it.

Even if you are giving symptomatic treatment, taking palliative measures in an emergency to alleviate some distress, perhaps using some well-tried formula for this purpose — never neglect the pulses. Even if you are not 'acting on the pulse signs', see what the pulses have to say. In this way you will learn how the pulses alter in response to what you do.

The pulses will tell you not only whether an organ is hyper- or hypo-active, or has excess or deficiency of energy, etc.; they will also tell you whether an organ is physiologically full or empty. This you should test on yourself, and on anyone else you can. Read the Bladder pulse before and after urination. Read the Large Intestine pulse before and after an evacuation. Read the Stomach pulse before and after a meal.

One practitioner of my acquaintance told me, with a certain amount of self-satisfaction over his Chinese pulse-reading prowess, ''I can always find a deficiency on the Bladder Meridian — so I make it a rule to tone up the Bladder at the first treatment.'' Of course, he always found that — for the simple reason there was a toilet between the dressing room and his consulting room — patients seldom omitted to 'call in on the way'!

The Balancer Channel

You will recall, from our second lesson, that the Organ Meridians occur in pairs. Each Yin meridian is paired with a Yang meridian. You already have the list of these pairs. In the case of all the meridians, the Energy current flows out at or near the last point of the meridian and enters the first point of the meridian which follows it. The paired meridians have additional communicating channels which serve as ''balancers'' between the two meridians which form the pair.

For example: from the Heart meridian (I) a special communicating channel branches off to the Small Intestine (II). The point on the Small Intestine meridian where the flow through the 'balancer channel' from the Heart meridian enters it is called ''The Small Intestine Passage Point.'' There is also a 'balancer channel' from the Small Intestine meridian to the Heart meridian: where this channel enters the Heart meridian is the point known as ''The Heart Meridian Passage Point.''

This is to be carefully noted: the Passage point of a meridian is the name of the point where the Energy from its paired meridian comes in. It is at this point that the inflow, or overflow, may be controlled. This represents the traditional view of the Passage points. I will not confuse you by giving you details concerning the views of some European schools about the Passage points. Let it suffice that you be aware that there is some difference between the two schools over this — and, as one might expect, a corresponding difference in treatment technique at the Passage points.

The Passage points are among the most important acupuncture points on any meridian, and, therefore, they must be learned. Although so far in this Course we have not had the detailed list of points on all the meridians, it is expedient that we should have a complete list of the Passage points, though I shall not describe their positions yet.

BALANCER CHANNEL FOR ENERGY FLOW		POINT OF ENTRY (Passage Point)
From	To	At
I	II	II.7
II	I	I.5
V	VI	VI.5
VI	V	V.6
IX	X	X.6
X	IX	IX.7
III	IV	IV.4
IV	III	III.58
VII	VIII	VIII.5
VIII	VII	VII.37
XI	XII	XII.4
XII	XI	XI.40

In this Table you notice the meridians of the arm and the meridians of the leg have been arranged in their two groups. This will facilitate learning, for, by the end of the next Lesson, we shall have the six organ meridians of the arm completed in detail. It will also make it easier to begin our study of the Five elements, when the logic of the pairing will become plain.

Path & Points on the Lung Meridian (IX)

The first point on the Lung meridian you have already from the first lesson. All the same, I will describe it for you once more in terms of the A.U.M. It is two A.U.M. lateral to the mamelon line, and nearly 5 A.U.M. above the mamelon, in the first intercostal space. The second point (IX.2) is vertically above the first point, just under the clavicle in the small hollow where the sub-clavian artery may be felt pulsating. There should be no difficulty in placing this point.

IX. LUNGS MERIDIAN

Anterior Upper Arm

.2
.1

Upper extremity of
anterior ancillary crease

x.

- - - Deltoid "V"

.3

.4

.... Elbow fold

.5

.6

▲ = FORBIDDEN TO MOXA

.7
.8
.9

- - - - Wrist fold

.10

.11

.7

.8

.9

.10

.11

LUNGS MERIDIAN IX
POINTS: .7-.11

The meridian path goes down the midline of the brachial biceps. The third point is 1 A.U.M. below the level of the Deltoid V, or 6 A.U.M. above the elbow fold. This point is forbidden to moxa. There are no points on this meridian forbidden to the needle, but four of them are forbidden to moxa. The fourth point is 1 A.U.M. below the third point, or 5 A.U.M. above the elbow fold.

The fifth point, IX.5, is exactly where the path of the Lung meridian crosses over the elbow fold, just lateral to the brachial biceps tendon of insertion. From here, the path follows the median border of the supinator longus, between the supinator longus and the flexor carpi radialis, as far as its insertion on the radius. The sixth point is 5 A.U.M. from the elbow fold (7 A.U.M. from the wrist fold).

The path now follows the radial groove and the next three points are on the radial artery. IX.9 is on the wrist fold, IX.8, which is forbidden to moxa, is 1 A.U.M. proximal to the wrist fold, and IX.7 is 2 A.U.M. proximal to the wrist fold. Check these with your Chart.

The tenth point is to be found on the palmar aspect of the hand, just below the head of the first metacarpal, on the vertical thumb flexion fold (see Chart): this point is forbidden to moxa.

The eleventh and last point is at the thumb nail root, the internal ungueal angle (first finger side). This is also forbidden to moxa. Some authorities place this last point at the other corner of the thumb nail, i.e., the external ungueal angle.

Path & Points on the Large Intestine Meridian (X)

The Meridian of the Large Intestine, X, begins on the index finger at the root of the finger nail (thumb side) external ungueal angle. It goes towards the back of the hand following the external dorsal aspect of the forefinger. The second point is just distal, and the third point just proximal, to the metacarpo-phalangeal articulation of the index finger.

The fourth point, X.4, one of the really great points of acupuncture, is in the angle formed by the two first metacarpals (see Chart). This point is easy to locate, as is also the next, the fifth point (X.5), which is in the centre of the hollow known as the anatomical snuff box, at the level of the dorsal wrist flexure (see Chart).

We have A.U.M. divisions to locate points of the meridians travelling down the anterior of the arm; so, too, we have similar A.U.M. divisions to locate the points on the meridians travelling up the posterior aspect of the arm. Wrist fold to Elbow fold = 12 A.U.M.

Point X.11 is at the external extremity of the elbow fold, when the elbow is in full flexion.

The meridian pathway, from the wrist, goes up the postero external border of the extensor communis digitorum, and, about 3 A.U.M. from the elbow fold, it crosses over the extensor carpi radialis and supinator longus to the external extremity of the elbow fold. Having drawn this line, we now measure the spacing in A.U.M. from the wristfold. At 3 A.U.M. from the wristfold is point number six, X.6; the next four points are 1 A.U.M. apart from each other, i.e. at 7, 8, 9 and 10 A.U.M., respectively, are the points X.7, X.8, X.9 and X.10. (Some charts show X.7 as only 6 A.U.M. up from the wristfold, but one has to bear in mind that the placing will, at times, depend upon the position in which the limb is depicted.) One needs to remember that the fingers will detect a small depression, at the site of the acupuncture point in fleshy parts, formed by muscle or tendon crossings.

Our reference points for the posterior of the arm are the elbow fold level (just below the external condyle of the humerus) and the upper extremity of the posterior axillary fold. The distance between these two points is 9 A.U.M. Point number twelve, X.12, is 2 A.U.M. up, and point number thirteen, X.13, is 3 A.U.M. up from the elbow fold. X.13 is forbidden to moxa.

The path follows the triceps to the deltoid V, at 7 A.U.M., and here is point number fourteen, X.14.

The line now goes to the external of the acromio-clavicular articulation, "the point of the shoulder." Where the path touches the acromion, between the head of the humerus and the acromion, is the fifteenth point, X.15. If the arm is raised sideways, a small hollow is formed at this site — the acupuncture point is in the middle of this hollow. The sixteenth point, X.16, is internal to the acromio clavicular articulation. See Chart.

From here the path crosses obliquely over the sterno-cleido-mastoidus to the anterior of the angle of the lower jaw. Point number seventeen, X.17 is just behind the sterno-cleido-mastoidus, and point eighteen 1 A.U.M. vertically above point 17.

The nineteenth and twentieth points are near the nose. X.19 is 1/2 A.U.M. from the mid-line of the naso labial furrow (called by artists "the gutter"), halfway between the upper edge of the top lip and the nostril.

The last point, X.20, is in the small depression which can be felt at the upper part of the naso-genion crease. You will know soon enough when you are "on" this point, as it is usually quite painful to press, and often will make the eyes water. Both these last points (.19 and .20) are forbidden to moxa.

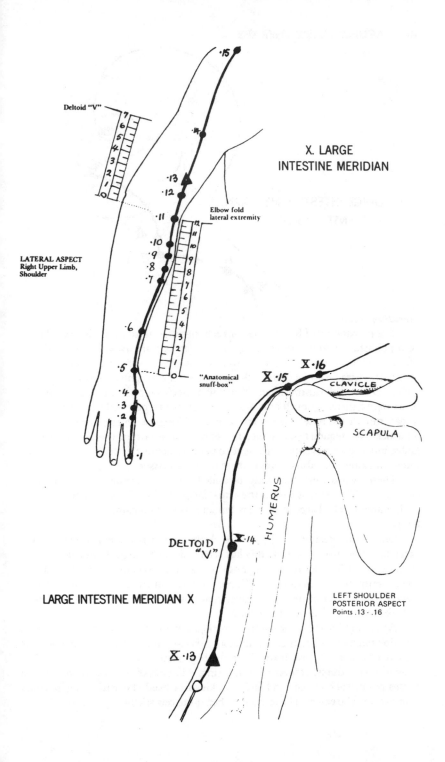

Deltoid "V"

X. LARGE
INTESTINE MERIDIAN

Elbow fold
lateral extremity

LATERAL ASPECT
Right Upper Limb,
Shoulder

"Anatomical
snuff-box"

CLAVICLE

SCAPULA

HUMERUS

DELTOID
"V"

LARGE INTESTINE MERIDIAN X

LEFT SHOULDER
POSTERIOR ASPECT
Points .13 - .16

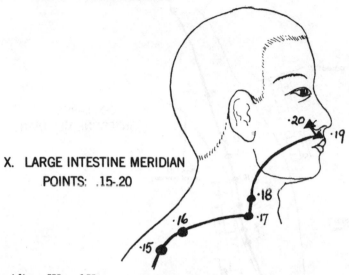

X. LARGE INTESTINE MERIDIAN
    POINTS: 15-20

Meridians IX and X

The preparation of Repertories for each meridian separately has never before been published in any Western language, as far as I am aware. This is a pity, because following this plan certain facts about the meridians are revealed that might otherwise take a lot of unearthing from a full and comprehensive Repertory which included all the meridians. You will notice that on meridians IX and X a great many throat, mouth and nose troubles are treatable. They have special throat, mouth and nose troubles are treatable. These two meridians have special influence over tegumentary tissue, not only surface skin of the body, face and limbs, but also wherever the tegument comes into contact with air (such as in the throat and lungs) but also wherever there is mucous tissue.

These two organs may aptly be called "slime" organs. Both deal with elimination. The skin, as well as the actual large intestine, is an important organ of elimination. The Large Intestine is but an involuted tegument; as are also the lungs.

One of the greatest of all points in Acupuncture is the fourth point of the Large Intestine meridian, X.4: this has been called The Great Eliminator. X.4 is included in a wide variety of 'couplings' or 'special combinations' of points for specific purposes. If I were asked, "If one wished to memorize one point only, is there any one point of such importance that you would choose it?" — there is little doubt in my mind I would go for X.4.

As a single point it can be used to regularize and tone up the entire large intestine function: also, as an eliminator, it is used to control the elimination of mental as well as physical toxins from the organism. It is useful in fevers when there is intense thirst, or fever with shivering. All kinds of skin conditions respond to this point, such as acne and boils: all kinds of headache arising out of faulty elimination. The effect on headaches is often quite remarkable.

You will also realize there is a wide range of pains in the upper part of the body, in the neck, chest and limbs, eyes, sinuses, teeth, etc., amenable to treatment at X.4: also, inflammation of eyelids and conjunctiva, mouth, lips, tonsils, nose, etc.

X.4 is also diagnostically quite useful. If you place your thumb well into the point X.4 and your middle finger opposite to it in the palm, near the thenar eminence, so that your thumb and finger serve as pincers, you will, by working the finger and thumb about, be able to feel the condition of the tissues. If, for example, it feels as if there were a rubbery lump inside, or a small sausage-shaped lump inside, deep in the tissues, you would know that the congested, bound-up, unfree condition here mirrors the state of the actual colon. If the flesh between your finger and thumb feels limp or toneless, it will be but a reflection of the large intestine lack of tonicity.

If we can alter the condition of the deep tissues at X.4 by massage, and bring them back to a living, pliable, supple condition, free of congestions and adhesions, then whatever is achieved here will have comparable beneficial repercussions on the colon and the entire large intestine function. Regular use of this point is generally extremely beneficial.

Now for some special combinations of points, or couplings.

When children have such symptoms as cough, fever, breathing difficulty, or throat troubles of any kind, the combination of X.4, X.1 and IX.11 is especially useful. In adults, too, this can be used to relieve bronchitis. X.4 and X.11 is a combination that may be used for all afflictions of the head, face, eyes, and nose. X.2 is a special point for constipation. I have known a few moments' massage treatment at this point to bring about a good bowel movement within ten minutes; the patient was constipated, congested, and without urge immediately before the treatment. Actually I did this particular treatment in order to lower a temperature that, in my opinion, had been too high for too long and must be reduced. But think of X.2 primarily as a special point for constipation rather than fever. For all disorders involving trachea and throat the combination of X.11 and X.15 may safely be used with good effects expected. The combination of X.4, IX.11 and IX.9 has particular influence over the mouth. In the Common Cold, think of X.19 and X.20.

You will notice from an examination of the repertories you have been given so far that some local conditions are treated locally; and some internal or distant conditions are treated near the extremities. Gradually several pictures will begin to form in your mind — we shall be sorting some of these pictures out soon in subsequent lessons when we come to discuss principles used to guide the practitioner in the choice of points to treat. In the meantime, see what you are able to observe and deduce for yourself.

With regard to repertories, do bear in mind, always, that NO repertory, however extensive, can ever include all possible combinations of symptoms, conditions and circumstances. Repertories are, at best, general guides.

5

The Three-Heater Meridian (VI)

The twelve internal organs of traditional acupuncture include the organs not recognized as such by Western physiologists. The organ known as "the circulation" or "vaso-constrictor" does not really represent much difficulty for the Western student, for he can well visualize the whole circulation system of blood vessels being looked upon as an organ, even though it is not neatly located in a relatively small space such as the heart, but is diffused throughout the whole organism.

The organ known as "the three-heater," "thermo-regulator," "three foci," "three burning spaces" and many other variants, does, however, represent difficulty for many students. Whereas it is easy for us to accept the fact of temperature maintenance and regulation, visualization is not easy without a picture of an actual location of specialized tissues.

Before I go on to describe the path of the meridian of the three-heater, I consider it advisable to spend some time trying to give you sufficient information about the organ to enable you to get a clear and satisfactory mental picture. It is no good if we only memorize the label attached to an organ, and still have no clear idea as to just where the label belongs. After all, when one treats a patient it is flesh and blood one is treating, not labels!

If we are going to look for an organ, or specialized tissue, that could correspond to the three-heater, we might just as well form as clear a picture as we can about what such an organ should do: and then look in the most likely place for these requirements to happen. We are going to look for a three-heater; let us, therefore, think and classify in terms of three.

Thermo-regulation involves three distinct, though co-ordinated, functions. First, the temperature must be registered somewhere, or be sensed. Secondly, variations either side of a set norm must "trigger off" the regulators, and, thirdly, processes must operate to bring about the required effects.

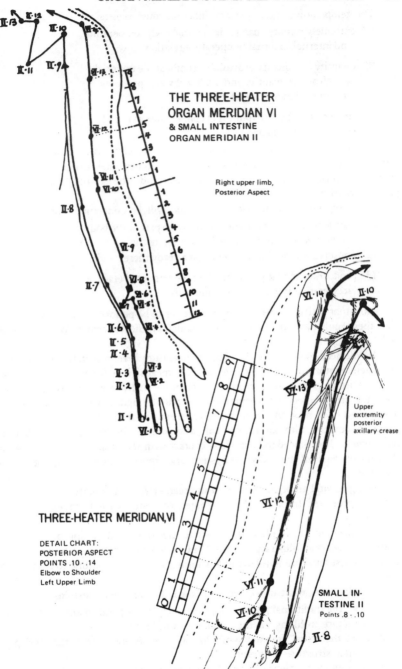

THE THREE-HEATER
ÓRGAN MERIDIAN VI
& SMALL INTESTINE
ORGAN MERIDIAN II

Right upper limb,
Posterior Aspect

THREE-HEATER MERIDIAN,VI

DETAIL CHART:
POSTERIOR ASPECT
POINTS .10 - .14
Elbow to Shoulder
Left Upper Limb

Upper
extremity
posterior
axillary crease

SMALL IN-
TESTINE II
Points .8 - .10

The temperature/organ sensory function must register:

(1) extremely minute changes in internal body temperature, and internal/external temperature relationships;

(2) quantity and quality of available combustible material, as well as the quantity and quality of waste products of combustion in the system;

(3) efficiency of the distribution of combustible material and waste elimination.

The temperature/organ regulatory function amounts to an automatic self-regulating co-ordination of three master or key switches: one 'triggered by heat', another 'triggered by chemical reaction', and the third 'triggered by pressure/rhythm'.

The temperature/organ effector function will be concerned with

(1) transfer of heat or heat-energy from one part of the body to another — either to retard or accelerate this;

(2) conservation or dissipation of heat already there; and

(3) production of heat within the body — either to retard or accelerate this process of manufacture.

Now that we have three sets of three duties to be performed, let us see where all of these could have their one sensory/regulatory/effector centre. Where must it be?

It will need to be where the blood temperature is representative of the total blood temperature of the inner organs. This means, it will have to be in close contact with an artery, and, in order to get an optimally representative picture of the whole arterial blood's oxygenated chyle content (qualitative and quantitative), it will need to be near an artery not too far removed from the heart. The fact of being in contact with an artery will also satisfy the beat/pressure/rhythm requirement. It will need to be in close contact with the brain, in particular with the control centre of the endocrine system, and, therefore, on an artery going to the brain.

Being so vital an organ — if such an organ exists — it will need to be almost perfectly protected from all risk of trauma or disturbance from external circumstances.

The diagram I have drawn to illustrate the traditional placing of the three-heater is based on an illustration to the Nei Ching. I have made no attempt to copy all the Chinese lettering, but have only shown enough of the outline to convey the idea.

Now let us see what answer we get to the following three questions

(1) Does the traditional position approximately correspond to any anatomical structure fulfilling all the conditions outlined?

(2) Does the actual drawing symbolize with reasonable clarity that this particular structure is meant?

(3) Does modern science in the West confirm this?

THE THREE-HEATER
THERMO-REGULATION SENSE ORGAN

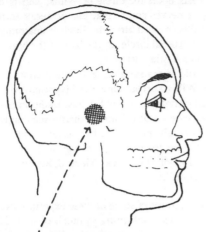

LOCATION OF THE "CIRCLE OF
WILLIS" FOR COMPARISON
WITH TRADITIONAL CHINESE
LOCATION, SEE ILLUSTRATION
BELOW.

府 焦 三 陽 少 手

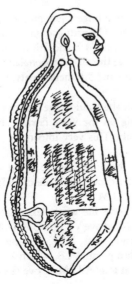

THE THREE BURNING SPACES
Rough sketch of a reproduction
from the Ling Shu Wen Chich Yas

In answer to these three questions:

(1) The position in the Chinese diagram closely approximates to that part of the hypothalamus which rests upon the circle of Willis, and is of the same tissue matrix as the optic nerves and retina, just posterior to the pituitary body. The Circle of Willis (named after the English anatomist who lived A.D. 1621-1675) is the arterial circle, at the base of the brain, formed by the internal carotids and basilar arteries;

(2) The Chinese drawing could be read as a crude representation of the internal carotids and circle of Willis surrounding the Hypothalamus;

(3) Western medical scientific confirmation of Far East tradition has been made by the discovery of the existence of a ''human thermostat'' at the exact site indicated. The discovery results principally from experiments conducted by Dr. T. H. Benzinger (and his team) as head of the calorimetry branch and the bio-energetics division of the Naval Medical Research Institute in Bethesda, Maryland, U. S. A.

In 1961, when I read an account of some of these experiments, I was indeed encouraged to find Western science confirming so much of what I had accepted years before through the study of Tibetan and other Far East medicine/philosophy.

It is of especial interest to us in acupuncture that the heart, small intestine, circulation, and three-heater are all classified as fire organs. We shall be hearing more of this when, in the next lesson, we begin our study of the Five Elements.

Paths & Points on the Three-Heater Meridian

This meridian has its first point on the ring finger, just proximal and lateral to the internal ungueal angle (little-finger side). The path goes up the inner border of the ring finger passing between the heads of the 4th and 5th metacarpals. The second point, VI.2, is between the knuckles at the metacarpophalangeal articular line. The third point, VI.3, is between the 4th and 5th metacarpals, just proximal to the heads of the metacarpals.

The path then goes over the dorsum of the hand to the centre of the dorsal wrist flexure, the fourth point, VI.4, being on the wrist flexure, between the heads of the ulna and radius and the carpals. This very important point is forbidden to moxa.

The reference points we now take are these: the centre of the dorsal wrist flexure and, at the elbow (as for the other meridians already described), the elbow fold, the distance being reckoned as 12 A.U.M.

The fifth point, VI.5, is 2 A.U.M. above the wrist flexure, between the radius and ulna. The sixth point is one A.U.M. above VI.5 (or 3 A.U.M. from the wrist flexure), close to the radius; the seventh point, VI.7, is at the same level, but on the ulna border (see chart). The eighth point, VI.8, which is forbidden to the needle, lies between the ulna and radius at four A.U.M. above the dorsal wrist flexure.

Try to get a clear picture in your mind of this three-heater meridian path —
and remember that, with the arm in the anatomical position, the path on reaching
the sixth point turns at a right angle inwards (towards the body) to the seventh
point, and then outwards and upwards at an acute angle to the eight point.

The ninth point, VI.9, is 7 A.U.M. up from the dorsal wrist flexure, in the
centre line between the radius and ulna. The meridian goes over the olecranon, in
the olecranon fossa and up the posterior of the arm on the brachial triceps tendon,
then between the long and lateral heads of the triceps to the deltoid, and up to the
postero-external tip of the acromion.

Our reference points covering the path from the elbow to the shoulder will
be: the elbow fold (which is at the same level as the olecranon) and the lateral tip
of the acromion; between these two reference points are 12 A.U.M.

The tenth point, VI.10, which is in the olecranon fossa, is at the lateral
border of the triceps tendon. It will be found at one A.U.M. above the elbow fold
line. The eleventh point, VI.11, is one A.U.M. above the tenth point. See chart.

The twelfth point, VI.12, is five A.U.M. above the elbow fold. At nine
A.U.M. above the elbow fold or three A.U.M. below the acromion is the thirteenth point, VI.13. The fourteenth point, VI.14, is at the level of the acromion
in the small hollow which forms on raising the arm. See detail chart for locating
points 12, 13 and 14 on page 51.

The fifteenth point, VI.15, is on the trapezius muscle (median postero-
superior of the shoulder) about half-way between the point of the shoulder and the
base of the neck. I have drawn a special diagram to show this exact location, as this
is an important point indicated in all conditions aggravated by cold and damp
weather. I give further instructions to locate it exactly: follow these on the detail
diagram on page 57.

Draw a horizontal line through the tip of the spinous process of the second
dorsal vertebra. Draw a vertical line touching the inner border of the scapula. Call
the distance between the spinous process of D.1 and the point where the
horizontal and vertical lines cross AB. Extend the horizontal line laterally 1/2
AB. This then locates VI.15 exactly. It is usually found to be quite painful under
heavy digital pressure. This point is known as "The Hygrometric Point".

The path now goes to the mastoid process: the sixteenth point, VI.16,
forbidden to moxa, is behind the mastoid process posterior to the sterno-cleido-
mastoidus tendon. The seventeenth point, VI.17, is just anterior to the mastoid
process, under the ear lobe.

The detail diagram shows the location of points 18, 19, 20, 21, 22 and 23
which need no further description. The points VI.18 and VI.23 are forbidden to
moxa, and VI.19 and VI.20 are forbidden to the needle. All the points in the
neighborhood of the ear are important local points for the treatment of deafness.

Path & Points on the Small Intestine Meridian (II)

The path of this organ meridian begins, as you will recall, with its first point close to the internal ungueal angle of the little finger. The path follows the line at the meeting of the dorsal and palmar skin, as far as the wrist. This line is clearly visible, especially on a coloured subject.

The second point, II.2, is just distal to the metacarpophalangeal articulation of the little finger; and the third point, II.3, just proximal to this articulation. The fourth point, II.4, is just proximal to the base of the fifth metacarpal (between the pyramidus and the fifth metacarpal).

The fifth point, II.5, is at the inner extremity of the dorsal wrist flexure, at the extremity of the styloid process of the ulna.

The path goes from the styloid process to the elbow, following the postero-internal border of the ulna, to the olecranon. Point number six, II.6, is one A.U.M. proximal to the styloid process, and the seventh point II.7 is five A.U.M. from the wrist flexure (styloid).

The eighth point, II.8, is at the level of the elbow flexure, at the postero internal of the elbow about 1/2 A.U.M. distal to the upper extremity of the olecranon process (known as the 'funny bone') on the ulnar nerve.

From the elbow the path follows up the medial part of the brachial triceps to the level of the upper extremity of the posterior axillary fold. The ninth point 11.9 is on the vertical extension of this axillary fold line, just below the scapulohumeral articulation. This point is forbidden to moxa.

A special detailed chart is drawn on page 81 to facilitate exact location of the next six points on this meridian.

The tenth point, II.10, is in the angle formed by the spine of scapula and the acromion. It will be found that this point is also on the vertical extension of the posterior axillary fold line. The eleventh point, II.11, is vertically below the broadest part of the spine of scapula at the horizontal level of the tip of the spinous process of the fifth dorsal vertebra. Point number twelve, II.12, is above the spine of scapula, in the supra-spinous fossa; and point thirteen, also in the supra-spinous fossa, is at the horizontal level of the spinous process of the third dorsal vertebra, vertically below VI.15.

The fourteenth point, II.14, is on the vertical line of the medial border of the scapula at the horizontal level of the tip of the spinous process of the first dorsal vertebra; and the fifteenth point, II.15, is on the trapezius at the horizontal level of the spinous process of the seventh cervical vertebra.

A careful study of the charts, and especially the detail charts, will make it relatively simple to locate these points. For the locating of these points I have followed with meticulous care the Chinese charts which are currently in use in China for locating acupuncture points. They agree in the main with the traditional placing as described by Dr. Wu Wei Ping.

It is understandable that these descriptions apply only if the subject is standing in the ''anatomical position''; once, however, you have a clear picture in your mind of the structures involved, the points can be located with the subject in any position.

Points sixteen to nineteen may most easily be found by referring to the charts and detail diagrams. Point number eighteen, II.18, is forbidden to moxa.

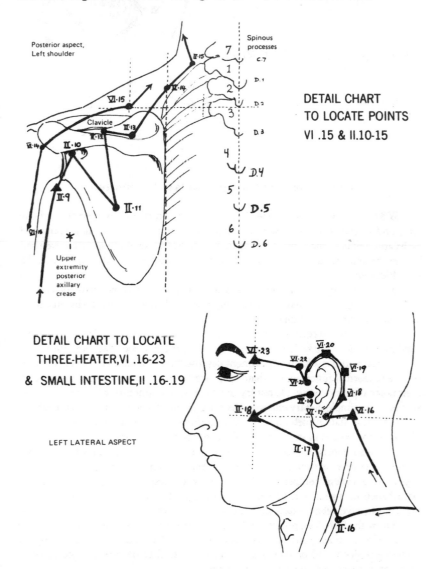

DETAIL CHART
TO LOCATE POINTS
VI .15 & II.10-15

DETAIL CHART TO LOCATE
THREE-HEATER,VI .16-23
& SMALL INTESTINE,II .16-.19

LEFT LATERAL ASPECT

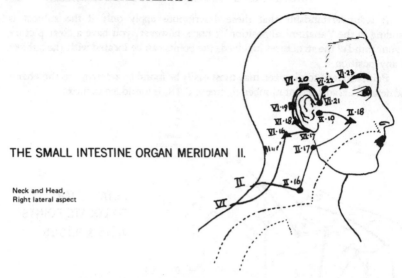

THE SMALL INTESTINE ORGAN MERIDIAN II.

Neck and Head,
Right lateral aspect

Limitations and Forbidden points of Acupuncture

We have now completed the detailed description of the six meridians of the arm, and in the next few lessons we shall be having a rest from descriptions of paths and points of the remaining organ meridians (those of the leg), for we shall be turning our attention to the actual forms of treatment at the points, and the Five Elements.

Before one begins treatment of any kind it is well to know what the contra-indications might be. There are relatively few, and most of them obvious commonsense contra-indications.

First, we should recognize the *limitations* of acupuncture, and not try to treat conditions which clearly do not come within the proper scope of acupuncture.

Acupuncture is a form of treatment designed to re-balance vital energy and to restore to normal functioning whatever processes may have become disturbed in their normal performance. Do not try to adjust by acupuncture what can better be arrived at by simple dietary changes. Bear this in mind when dealing with a patient in an extreme state of debilitation, for acupuncture is not a means of supplying energy to the system in the way that adequate nourishment and rest will do.

It is also common sense that one would not treat a person who is drunk unless, of course, action is taken to sober him. Again, it is not suitable to treat anyone in a violent temper, or in any extreme state of emotional excitement, disturbance or stress. Under the foregoing conditions the pulses could not be expected to give reliable data in respect to deep-rooted vital energy imbalances.

Know the forbidden points, and to what action they are forbidden.

A Master of acupuncture may take all kinds of liberties: but until one has been in practice for 15 or 20 years one would do well to observe the prohibitions with the utmost and most scrupulous care.

Never use needles at any acupuncture point on a pregnant woman.

Do not use needles on the cranial points of an infant. In general, as regards treatment of infants, it would be well to confine action at acupuncture points to massage treatment; this applies also to the very aged.

Never insert a needle into a tumour: it is better to apply this rule to any swelling.

Never insert a needle elsewhere than into acupuncture points. Acupuncture treatment is given at acupuncture points and only at these points.

The following organ meridians must not be allowed to bleed: I, IV, VI, VII, XI, XII.

By tradition, it is considered useless to insert needles for the purpose of acupuncture treatment if the environment temperature exceeds blood heat. The reason for this will become clear when we go further into the details of actual needle work.

Although not expressly forbidden, it is wise to avoid treatment immediately following a meal: allow from one hour after a light meal to five or six hours after a very heavy meal.

If one bears in mind that the Vital Energy is of an 'electrical nature', then one would naturally not use acupuncture treatment if the atmospheric electrical balance is disturbed, such as occurs during thunderstorms, or even in gales and high winds. The Chinese teach that one should not treat with acupuncture at full moon; nor in any environmental condition or phenomena associated with the moon, namely near the sea during spring high tides.

There is a contra-indication that never seems to occur to the Western mind; but is, nevertheless, of great importance in acupuncture, namely: a practitioner who is not in good health should not treat a patient. This is reasonable on at least two counts: in the first place, the standard or norm by which to assess the patient is no longer itself normal — for the practitoner's heart beat, pulse rate, respiration rate, etc., should represent the norm. In the second place, a disturbed vital energy in the practitioner could re-act unpredictably upon the patient and the treatment either becomes ineffective or detrimentally aggravates the patient's disturbance.

There are certain conditions and circumstances, probably not foreseen by the Ancients, but which, nevertheless, logically follow from their general rule of avoiding acupuncture action if the atmosphere is electrically disturbed; such conditions might arise in the proximity of radio installations or power generating stations of some kinds. If there is any doubt in the practitioner's mind, he would do well to follow the traditional Yorkshire adage, "If in doubt, do nowt."

There are certain health hazards that will undoubtedly come to the fore fairly soon, such as those consequent on very high speed travel, and, of course, space travel. It is early yet to know whether acupuncture will provide a suitable treatment for space-age disorders or not. Personally, I think that unless an adequate understanding of the vital energy concept is attained, there is every chance that Western medicine will not be able to deal with the very diseases and disturbances Western science creates.

Points of Restricted Action

Meridian	Forbidden to MOXA	Forbidden to NEEDLE	Bleeding
Heart		I. 2	I. Forbidden
Small Intestine	II. 9,18		
Bladder	III. 1,2,5,6,30,50,51, 54,62.	III. 1&2 pique superficially with extreme caution; wiser to avoid. III. 16,56.	III. 54 can be piqued to bleed a few drops for vomiting & diarrhea.
Kidneys		IV. 1 use only in absolute necessity; extremely painful. IV. 11	IV. Forbidden
Circulation			V. 3 made to bleed for vomiting & diarrhea.
Three-Heater	VI. 4,16,18,23.	VI. 8,19,20.	VI. Forbidden
Gall	VII. 1,15,22,33,42.	VII. 3,18.	VII. Forbidden
Liver		VIII. 12	
Lungs	IX. 3,8,10,11.		
Large Intestine	X. 13,19,20.		
Stomach	XI. 1 use joss stick only, 7,8,9,17 (nipple) 36 to children under 7 years of age	XI. 1,9,17 (nipple) Points 2 to 19 inc. to be piqued superficially	XI. Forbidden
Spleen	XII. 1,7,9	XII. 1 & 2 during pregnancy 11 pique with caution (on femoral artery)	XII. Forbidden
Conception Vessel	Conc. 1 3 & 4 if Bladder is full 8 unless first filled with salt (umbilicus) 22 to children under 7 years of age	Conc. 8,17 22 pique just in skin only with extreme caution (Adam's Apple) 22 to children under 7 years of age	
Governor Vessel	Gov. 6,7,15,16,17,18,25	Gov. 7,10,11,17,24	Gov. 7 & 17 forbidden

Note that XI. 17 and Gov. 7 & 17 are totally prohibited to all action.

Part two

THE FIVE ELEMENTS AND ACUPUNCTURE TECHNIQUES

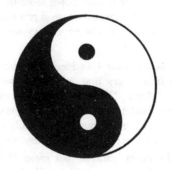

6

The Five Elements

We leave the study of the Organ Meridians and the points on their paths for the time being, and turn our attention to the Five Elements. In this Lesson it is our aim to try and build up a clear and simple picture of the general principles involved, and to relate the Five Elements to the Twelve Pulses, and so on.

These Medicine-philosophic principles provide us with 'tools', or means of appreciating whether or not a therapeutic problem exists; what is its nature; what means have we at hand to solve it, and so on. Time devoted to the theoretical aspect will indeed not be wasted time. It is all very well to memorize a number of special Formulae — or to have an extensive Repertory to which to refer — but there are many cases that do not fit neatly into one or other 'formula pigeon-hole'. Only an understanding of Principles will help us to solve many individual differences. As practitioners, it is the actual 'down-to-earth' operational aspect that matters, and we shall, therefore, concentrate upon practical application of Theory at the earliest possible moment — but some Theory we must have as our basis.

When we start to talk about the Five Elements, *Wood, Fire, Earth, Metal, Water,* yet in the same breath, say that, of course, we do not refer to actual 'Wood', 'Fire', 'Earth', 'Metal', 'Water', we must be prepared to be accused of talking nonsense from the outset. As the Five Elements will be referred to so often, and will be used so much in the course of our daily work, they have just got to mean something to us that does not appear as nonsense.

If we call them "Elements" and do not mean "elements", what do we mean? They are symbols of "five stages of change", the Chinese phrase for which has been incorrectly translated as the "Five Elements". To know this helps us in trying to understand Chinese thought concerning the principles underlying the phenomena of the physical world.

According to Far Eastern Tradition—that is, the Tradition that concerns us now in this text—the Cosmos as we know and experience it at the present day had, in the dim remote past, a Beginning.

This Beginning lies beyond the physical and is described in such terms as the Unmanifest, the Undifferentiated, the Inchoate, the First Cause—words attempting to express Something that cannot be imagined; a state of inactivity where there is No Process, No Thing. We take it as axiomatic that something new can be made only out of what is there. Since we have no material thing, then all things, processes, etc. must derive or be made from "That which is already there". Moreover, the agency or power must also be "That which is already there."

So, out of Itself and by Itself the First Cause makes Itself manifest by the Primary Act of Self-Assertion or Self-Positing. Assertion implies its opposite— Negation. Thus with the first assertion or POSITIVE, simultaneously there occurs the first negation or NEGATIVE. The two Poles are born together as antagonists that are, at the same time, complementary.

Through various stages (cosmologically speaking) of dynamic interplay of these two polarities, a series of focussing, condensations, crystallizations, etc., take place—until we arrive at the Totality of complex aggregates that we experience as the present-day world.

The various stages have been named according to some characteristic.

We need to remember that there are several Far Eastern versions, e.g. Indian, Tibetan, Chinese, Mongolian, etc. We find that though they may differ in detail, emphasis, nomenclature, and so on, the underlying Principles appear to run parallel.

Sometimes we find the emphasis placed upon Duality, sometimes upon Trinity, or upon Four, Five, or more divisionings. I do not intend to dwell in the maze of Orders of abstraction; it is enough for our purpose to realize there is such a maze. We shall not get lost in it so long as we keep reminding ourselves that Concepts exist as postulates of the Human Mind. We accept certain postulates as a matter of convention in order to explain certain phenomena. The Concepts that we find useful in Acupuncture for the purpose of explaining, classifying, and so on, are quite simple.

Everything that exists has a Beginning. We refer to the 'beginning' as the Stage of Minimum existence.

There is also a Stage of Maturity or Maximum existence.

The transition from minimum to maximum, and then from maximum to minimum, represents the fundamental rhythm or cycle in nature.

But it is no sudden rise from the minimum to the maximum; nor sudden fall from maximum to minimum. The nature of Change is process, not catastrophe.

An example of this rhythmic process is illustrated diagrammatically using as our example the growth of a plant. This represents a very simplified instance of a 'Life-Cycle'. Very simple, but do not be misled by this simplicity. I might add, this apparently childish simplicity.

I have illustrated diagrammatically another example, that of the yearly rhythm in a tree, whose 'life cycle' may extend over many, many years.

In these instances of cycles, one should, I feel, consider them rather more in the nature of a spiral than as a 'flat' closed circle.

You will readily appreciate the logic of the statement that each Stage

A Natural Cycle
(Plant Growth)

```
LIGHT        +     MAXIMUM
_____   Ground Level
XXXXXXXXXXXXXXXXXXXXXXXXXXXXX
XXXXXXXXXXXXXXXXXXXXXXXXXXXXX
          XXXXXXXXX
DARK      XXXX  – XXX MINIMUM
          XXXX    XXX
XXXXXXXXXXXXXXXXXXXXXXXXXXXXX
```

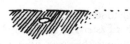

STAGE 1. Below the ground a seed or plant in a state of minimum, just prior to the first stirrings into activity.

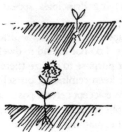

STAGE 2. In Spring the young shoot shows above ground and strives upward toward light and air. (Growth towards maturity.)

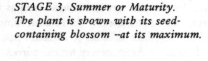

STAGE 3. Summer or Maturity. The plant is shown with its seed-containing blossom --at its maximum.

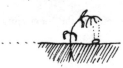

STAGE 4. Late Summer. Decrease or withdrawal of life begins when the seed is ripe for gathering or falls to the ground.

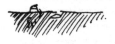

STAGE 5. Autumn. The season of gathering, storing (or the seed buried). This is the state of balance.

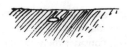

AS STAGE 1. Finally, in Winter once more the minimum, the new seed lies dormant ready for the coming Spring, when the cycle begins and fulfills itself all over again. This is known as the stage of the Power of Emptiness.

engenders the one which follows it, and each also foreshadows, with a controlling influence over, later stages. It is obvious, for example, that upon this year's harvest the success of next year's spring growth will depend.

The more complex the form of life, the more of these rhythmic cyclic processes are to be found taking place, at different speeds, with different cycle durations, on various levels, interweaving, intermingling, influencing each other, and being influenced by them. Whether the cycle completes itself in a few moments, hours, days, months or years, the Ancients considered the Stages of Change to conform to One Basic Pattern.

Though some cosmogonies enumerate nine stages, eight, or less, it seems that all agree that the number of States is, in final analysis, reducible to Five. A name has been given to each stage. At the present day the names by which these Stages are known are the names of the five Elements: Water, Wood, Fire, Earth, Metal.

Exactly how and why the Ancients came to settle upon these five names, I do not know.

These five names should not be looked upon as names of substances or things but as process Stages, or Powers.

Using a little imagination we are able to find a logical sequence from Water to Wood, Wood to Fire, Fire to Earth, and Earth to Metal. Thus, the presence of Water makes Plant Life possible; Water fosters and engenders Wood (or Plant Life); Wood serves as fuel for Fire; Water controls Fire, in that it will extinguish it. Among these Elements, logical and reasonable connections are easy to find.

Fire can be said to engender Earth in that fire makes ashes. Various links can be found between the Elements as they follow one upon the other. These links may be found on one level or another, as, for example, in the formation of a heavenly body: the glowing ball of fire which condenses to form a crust, or shall we say there is a crystallization to Earth from Fire. In order to make our links, we need to keep our minds switching, as it were, from one level to another.

Earth, especially in its fecundity, is controlled by Plant Life, through natural decomposition, etc. Or, looked at from another angle, Earth can be subjected by Wood by means of sharpened sticks, the primitive tools of husbandry.

As regards Earth engendering Metal, our difficulties begin. We can, of course, trace a logical sequence between Metal Ore and Earth. Earth (ore) can, in this respect, be said to produce Metal. It is also clear that Fire controls or subjects Metal by melting it.

It is not so easy to interpret "Metal gives Birth to Water", though we are able easily enough to appreciate that Metal may be said to control or subject Wood, for metal implements cut wood, or control Plant Life. The Control influence need not, however, be always destructive.

In calling Mythology to my aid, I well realize that I may be handing out ready-made ammunition for the use of those critics who deride Far East Medicine philosophy, or who, indeed, poke fun at anything that goes beyond the bonds of what is measurable by modern scientific instruments. Nevertheless, I, personally, found what appears to me to be a satisfactory possible linkage which indicates that

Metal is, after all, a suitable label for this stage — the stage between Earth (solid) and Water (liquid) — and which provides a reasonable linkage of the two organs corresponding to Metal, namely, Lungs and Large Intestine.

According to one Far East myth, the World as we know it today presents a very different picture from what it once did. It now represents the outcome and

THE YEARLY RHYTHM OF A TREE

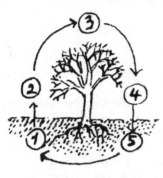

1. In winter, the sap lies dormant in the roots.

2. In spring, the sap level rises

3. and reaches the outer limits in summer, and

4. with the formation mature fruit in late summer, the receding or decrease begins.

5. Fruit and leaves fall in autumn, the sap recedes below the ground to lie in store for the cycle to begin once more at the proper time.

In connection with 'rising and falling' sap, it is not that the flow of sap changes from a flow upwards to a flow downwards; but rather that the height, to which the ever upward-flowing sap reaches, rises, and recedes.

THE FIVE BASIC ELEMENTS

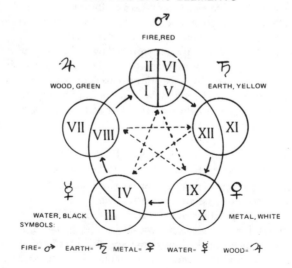

continuing manifestation of an unceasing warfare between the Devas and the Asuras (the angelic protagonists of Light and Darkness). Beings and things in the time before the Fall of the Asuras appeared and behaved very differently. For example, Metals were fluidic. The Food of the Gods was Golden. Food was taken in, used, and given up again unchanged. According to the Tibetan Chi-Schara-Badgan Medicine Philosophy, the present-day manifestation most closely resembling the golden nourishment of former time is the 'golden', relatively complete, nourishment of the egg yolk. In their fall the Asuras stole the food of the Gods, and took it down into the darkness, where it later evolved into the mucus and excrement producing organs. What was once a Mouth pointing upwards became the anus — a rectum. Relationship with the other orifices (nose, mouth, ears, eyes) is retained: this is clearly shown in Acupuncture by the fact that Points on the Colon or Large Intestine meridian are used to treat affections of mouth, nose, etc. Points on the Lung meridian are also often used to treat similarly in association.

The Lungs, organs once external in contact with Air, are now involuted, hidden in darkness, and mucosity; though they are still in direct contact with Air. The Colon is also an involuted skin organ, or air organ, producing mucus. Thus, the Metal Organs could as appropriately be referred to as the 'Slime' or mucus organs. A one-time fluidic metal now becomes Slime.

If we accept the notion of Slime, we are easily able to see how, by a process of filtration and separation, Slime (Metal) produces Water. The organs of filtration, the Kidneys, and those of liquid excretion, the Bladder and urethral canal, naturally follow on as the Water Organs. That the Water Organs control or subject the Fire Organs, Three-heater and Circulation, becomes obvious. Body temperature regulation is linked to Kidney and urinary Bladder function. Let us now leave this aspect and go back to the consideration of Basic Rhythm ''minimum to maximum, maximum to minimum.''

The fundamental notion is Polarization of a Unitary Force into Positive and Negative polarities; first, there is the predominance of Positive moving outwards from Nothing into Something (to full maturity), followed by decrease of Positive and predominance of Negative in the return movement to minimum.

I make no apologies for the time now being spent on this ''philosophical'' aspect, for I feel it will prove to be time well worth your while to try to get the 'feel' of Energy- and Polar-Activity Orientation. I shall try to illustrate the notions by a quick reference to the formation and movement of heavenly bodies, Sun and Planets — according, of course, to Far East cosmogony.

It is supposed that 'In the Beginning' there was a tensioning to a point of inequality in the undifferentiated Aether of Space, creating a focal point of Suction; or condensation to a Centre, together with Rotation. Thus, there was a Centripetal Urge, an urge inwards to a centre, and at the same time a balancing centrifugal Urge, an urge outwards from centre to periphery.

In this way a central Core or Sun, is formed, which becomes surrounded by a series of hollow globes, in layers somewhat like the skins and layers of an onion. The rotating hollow globes condense into planetary Rings which rotate with the

Sun (or Centre). These rings further condense until each consolidates to form a spherical planetary body.

Sun and Planet are related polarwise to each other. The Planet is both drawn towards the Sun by centripetal action, and repelled, away from the Sun, by centrifugal action. The Planet, itself, is bi-polar.

It is a peculiarity of planetary bodies that they change polarity, i.e. polarity predominance, by their own power.

For an appropriate time the polar relationships are such that the two bodies, Sun and Planet, are drawn together. The planet strives towards the Sun. But when the planet comes to within a certain distance from the Sun, the planet's polarity (relative to the Sun) changes. The period of attraction comes to an end, and is followed by a period of repulsion. The planet then moves away from the Sun until it reaches a certain distance, when, once again, its inner polarity changes and it is once more attracted towards the Sun. This is an illustration of Fu Hsi's Law, "Unlike poles attract one another; like poles repel one another."

Throughout the life of a Sun or Planet there is rhythmic movement towards, and away from, the center. The polar changes occur within certain distance limits. If we add to this movement the revolution round the Sun, it will be seen that the planetary Orbit is not circular but elliptical. *The Elliptical Orbit represents a basic pattern in nature.* We can observe examples in many happenings and processes.

Each planetary manifestation has, within itself, both poles, X+ and —. First, the one predominates, then the other. So is our basic pattern set, and we shall see later how this is carried out in the Meridian Energy.

Provided that the bi-polar energy undergoes the natural rhythmic changes at the proper times, at the proper speeds, strengths, etc., the Event, Being or Circumstance, System or Organization remains constant, then we say that it is living in health.

The balance of Negative and Positive urges has to be maintained within limits appropriate to that particular manifestation.

We now return to our example of the Tree and the Sap. The tree Sap, or life-blood of the tree, is considered as a planetary body related polarwise to Earth Centre. The limit of closeness to the centre is marked by the tips of the roots: and the outermost limit is marked by the extremities of the outer twigs. There is a seasonal rhythmic change of polarity: The Sap level rises and recedes in seasonal rhythm.

Here I should mention that an individual tree is looked upon Not as a complete planet but as part of a planet. The complete 'tree planet' is made up of all the trees of that kind on the whole earth surface, forming a broad ring (or double ring, one north and one south of the equator). The planetary "ring-wave" travels round the earth with a tide-like motion describing an elliptical orbit.

Plant life, i.e. all plant life, represents the totality of internally moved bodies: each individual member is bound to one location on the earth surface.

Animal life represents a different class of life, namely, Organic bodies moved throughout. Each member, or individual animal, having its own centre, to which its own periphery is polarwise related; in addition, of course, to being related polarwise to Earth's centre. In other words, these organic bodies have within themselves both Solar and Planetary manifestations. Animal life, being a higher, that is to say, more complete form of life than plants, includes within itself the lower forms, functions and activities.

In this context 'lower' and 'higher' are not in any way intended to mean 'more', or 'less', ethical, moral, or any other worth, but simply more complete.

In animal life, there are vegetative functions and processes side by side with animal functions and processes: but the lower functions are raised to a new level.

Plant life represents a micro-planet. Earth and (plant) planet together represent a micro-solar system.

Animal life represents a micro-solar system in each individual member.

Now, as regards Man. Man does not belong to the animal class of life. I feel this to be highly important for us in Acupuncture; so important, indeed, that I would like you to underline it heavily in red, and never, never forget it. This distinction is of immense therapeutic significance, for, quite apart from the new dignity thus accorded to Man, we shall be able to appreciate the inadequacy of drug and other experiements carried out upon animals and then attempting to apply the results to Man.

Man belongs to a different class of life and, therefore, requires a therapeutic approach appropriate to that class of life.

As I see it, Acupuncture does represent a possible therapeutic approach which is appropriate to Man. I use the term 'Acupuncture' in a very broad sense to represent the Traditional Far East medical approach.

Man embodies an additional characteristic which raises him to a higher (more complete) class than Animal. Each individual Human represents a Micro-cosm, and has within himself all the lower manifestations, processes, functions, etc., raised to a new level, in addition to his own Human Characteristic.

If the outcome of this Lesson, Section 1, is no more than a realization (deep conviction) of the True Status and Dignity of Human Beings, I shall be satisfied that my efforts will have been well rewarded.

The Tibetan Medicine Philosophy referred to earlier does recognize the human status, for it places Inorganic 'life' in the Badgan Mode; Organic life, plant and animal, in the Schara mode; and Man in the Chi mode. But we cannot go into this further in this Course.

The next Lesson will continue with the Five Elements Doctrine. Read, re-read and reflect, and be receptive to the 'feel' of this Far East Orientation.

To sum up so far:

(i) Life functions as a complex aggregate of bi-polar Energy rhythms or cycles;

(ii) The health, well-being and continued existence of the individual depend upon the maintaining of dynamic rhythmic balance of polarities;

(iii) Each class of life has its own characteristic, and embodies those of all lower forms, but raised to a new level.

How Acupuncture Techniques Work

The term, "Acupuncture" — which, quite literally, means 'pricking with a needle' — tends to be misleading. It gives the impression that the needle technique is the one and only. There are several ways of bringing about the desired effect. The three main methods are Massage, Moxa and Needle, all three of which are equally effective. I shall deal with each one of these in that order, beginning with Massage.

Let us try to form some sort of idea of what is going on in the body or what phenomena we are dealing with. What state, condition or process is it we seek to alter in some way?

So far I have not come across any explanation which is, to my mind, completely satisfying. It may be many, many years before a theory is put forward that will be capable of explaining apparent contradictions, and resolving problems whose solutions have, up to the present, eluded us.

Until some big advance is made in our knowledge, and until some startling and revolutionary theory is formulated, the most satisfactory basis upon which we can think and work is that the Vital Energy represents some form of 'Electricity-Nature' phenomenon. This does not mean to say that Vital Energy is electricity, but rather that its behaviour, responses, reactions, etc., are such as to indicate that a great deal of the Laws applying to the behaviour of electricity also apply to Vital Energy.

It also appears to me that the Vital Energy manifestations and the Traditional methods used to bring about Vital Energy changes are, in some way, closely linked with 'colloids' and 'colloidal behaviour'. I think it is in this direction we should look for a workable theory.

Colloidal Behavior

In order that you may thoroughly understand this basis, I shall have to go into the subject of 'colloidal behaviour'. This does not mean that we shall be wandering away from the subject of acupuncture, but rather that we shall be going more deeply into the matter than is customary among acupuncture teachers.

It is not enough that a student learn how to 'go through the motions' of a treatment technique; unless there is enough understanding of what is happening, sooner or later a practitioner will find himself faced with a problem of treatment to which no answer is to be found in any textbook — and only his own understanding of the basis will enable him to work out a solution.

If you would like to know more about ''colloids'' than is possible for me to set down in this Lesson, I suggest you read Dr. Marjorie Swanson's monograph Scientific and Epistemologic Backgrounds of General Semantics, which comprises a series of lectures on Electro-colloidal Structure (published by the Institute of General Semantics, Lakeville, Conn.) I have compiled this Lesson mainly from notes made when I read Dr. Swanson's lecture series in 1956.

You are not expected to memorize this section dealing with 'colloids': it is sufficient if you read it through and get a general feel of the subject.

If you take a piece of paper and cut it in halves — take one of these halves and halve it — then one of these and halve it again, and repeat the operation over and over again, halving ever smaller and smaller pieces, you will soon realize that there comes a point where you could no longer carry on this subdivision without the aid of delicate instruments. Eventually, you would reach a point where further subdivision is no longer possible without involving change of chemical character. You will have reached molecular size. Now, between the smallest visible particle and the molecule is the size range sometimes referred to as 'the twilight zone of matter'. It is within this range that 'colloidal behaviour' happens. A colloid occurs when very fine particles of one material are suspended in other media (which may be gaseous or liquid). The particles themselves may be gaseous, liquid or solid.

A simple form of colloid can be exemplified in an emulsion where we have droplets of, let us say, some oily matter suspended in a watery medium. With some emulsions the minute, oily droplets will remain in suspension more of less indefinitely; with some other emulsions the tendency for the oily droplets to coalesce and settle is such that the emulsion is very unstable.

Colloids occur not only as particles of solids or liquids in liquid media (emulsions); but also as particles of solid matter in gaseous media (smokes); and liquids in gaseous media (mists).

In every colloid there are two tendencies or phases. There is the tendency for the finely divided particles to repel one another and remain apart: there is the tendency for the particles to coalesce or join up with neighbouring particles. These two phases are known in colloidal chemistry as the Sol and Gel phases. The Sol phase labels the tendency to stay finely divided (or even increase the subdivision and suspension): the Gel phase labels the uniting into larger units with the eventual cessation of the 'colloid' state. A colloid is said to be dead when Sol has become irreversibly Gel.

We can consider these two tendencies as being the tendency to maximum subdivision, when the ratio of surface exposed to volume of material is so large that the surface electrical charges cause the particles to repel one another (like polarities repel one another) to a greater degree than the internal charges tend to unite. The tendency to minimum subdivision occurs when the energies tending to unite, coagulate, flocculate or precipitate, predominate.

All colloids are unstable; but some far more so than others. As the state moves to increase Gel the colloid is said to age. In some colloids this ageing process is reversible, and the changes take the form of changes in viscosity. Some changes are slow, some are rapid.

It is scientifically and generally accepted that *All Life happens only where there is protoplasm behaving colloidally*. In living structures, organisms, the colloids are extremely sensitive with enormous possibilities as regards potential stability, reversibility of phase, etc. One of the characteristics of Life is periodicity or rhythm; in other words, fluctuations between the predominance of the Sol and Gel phases.

All colloids, very much so living colloids, are electrically sensitive. Living systems depend for their rhythmic behaviour upon the chemically alterable film (suface tension film behaving as a membrane), which divides the electrically conducting phases. Living organisms can be described as film-bounded and partitioned irritable systems: which is to say, 'sensitive to electrical currents'.

There are several factors which can disturb or change colloidal balance (structure); that is to say, accelerate or retard one phase or another, as, for example, all known forms of radiant energy can affect or alter colloids.

In an organism living in health, the complex totality of manifold colloidal structures behave with appropriate periodicity and rhythm between certain phase limits. Any phase of any of the colloidal systems which goes beyond the appropriate limit (or fails to reach a limit within the proper time) will affect the health of the organism as a whole. Likewise, any factor, intrinsic or extrinsic, capable of altering colloidal behaviour, will have a marked effect, one way or another, upon the welfare of the organism.

I now briefly sum up so far:

Colloidal behaviour is exhibited by materials of a very fine subdivision which involves surface activities and electrical characteristics;

All life processes involve at least electrical currents;

Electrical currents and other forms of energy are able to affect the colloidal structures upon which our physical characteristics depend, i.e. they influence our bodies and our minds;

All life is characterized by protoplasm behaving colloidally.

As regards acupuncture treatment techniques, I feel convinced that, whether one uses needles, moxa, or massage, we are simply making therapeutic use of one or more of the factors able to alter colloidal equilibrium.

As we shall have to refer to the various factors. I now set them down clearly.

1. PHYSICAL

e.g. X-rays, Radium, Ultra-violet Rays, Light, Heat, Electricity, Cathode Rays; in fact, all forms of radiant energy.

2. MECHANICAL

e.g. Friction, Puncture, Pressure, Percussion, Sound and Ultrasonic frequencies.

3. BIOLOGICAL

Factors, such as microbes, parasites, etc., do not come into the therapeutic factors for our attention in this Course, but they should be considered when making a diagnosis.

4. CHEMICAL

e.g. Drugs, Poisons, and some Foods. We shall be considering this factor later on, when we come to the dietary application of the Five Elements Laws.

The Massage Techniques

As I have just said in the previous section, all the acupuncture techniques (needle, moxa, massage, etc.) make therapeutic use of one or more of the factors known to be able to change colloidal equilibrium. Thus, though there are several different massage techniques — they all have this in common, namely, the ability to accelerate, retard, or even reverse Sol/Gel phases.

Obviously, before massaging (or taking any acupuncture action) at an acupuncture point, there would have to be a clear indication that the point is the correct one at which to take action. This will have been ascertained by one or more of the diagnostic measures, pulses, abdominal, complexion diagnosis, symptoms, syndromes, etc. Furthermore, the point will have been accurately and precisely located — and only then is it to be treated in the correct polarity.

There are but two polarities for treatment. Let us have a note of the conditions or kinds of conditions requiring the same polarity treatment.

Excess energy, hypertonicity, hyperactivity, hypersecretion, pain, spasm, etc., require draining, dispersion, sedation, soothing, relaxing, calming, releasing, or Yin action. In the Nei Ching the expression used for this polarity of action is "Draining" but I may use any of the synonyms as whim or fancy suits me.

Deficiency of energy, hypotonicity, hypoactivity, hyposecretion, torpid, sluggish, paralytic states, etc., require toning, stimulating, supplying, activating, focussing, enlivening, vitalizing or Yang action. The Nei Ching refers to this polarity of treatment as Supplementing.

Since only two polarities of action are needed, all our massage movements will be designed to act in one or the other of these two polarities, Yin or Yang.

Massage Techniques include the following:-

(i)   Use of a special massage instrument or 'needle';
(ii)   Use of the finger-nail for either friction or pressure;
(iii) Use of the fingers for friction, pressure, movement;
(iv)   Use of the knuckles, elbows, for pressure and movement;
(v)   Use of the knuckles, elbows, toes, knees, and heel of the hand for percussion.

The traditional massage instrument is in the form of an ivory or bone needle, ending not in a point but in a ball. The essential characteristic of the instrument is that the head, or part which comes into contact with the patient's flesh, shall be of an electrically non-conducting (insulating) material, such as bone, ivory, ebony, bakelite, plastic, etc.

A light, rapid rubbing on a dry surface with such an instrument will cause a small static charge to build up which, upon attaining a certain magnitude, will discharge itself. It has been demonstrated with various electrical instruments that acupuncture points coincide with small areas of low electrical resistance (high conductivity), relative to the lower conductivity of the surrounding tissues. Hence, a charge built up in the neighbourhood of an acupuncture point will, upon discharging itself, be released into the point of lowest resistance. The static charge is extremely small, but it is this very minuteness that gives to it penetration power sufficient to reach inner organs. The bone needle is rubbed lightly and rapidly in a circular movement closely round the acupuncture point. This movement gives treatment of Yang polarity to supplement, tone up, stimulate, activate, etc. In lieu of a bone needle, I have, on occasion, used the plastic cap of my fountain pen, with immediate effect. It is not always the expensive-looking and elaborate piece of mechanism that is the most effective!

The opposite polarity of treatment to drain or disperse an excess or accumulated charge is by relatively slow, steady, firm circular movements of the same instrument starting closely round the point and gradually increasing in diameter to "spread" the charge and thus disperse it.

The Chinese practitioner would often use his fingernail in lieu of the bone needle, for the nail — being of itself a bony or horny substance — is electrically insulating. Provided the fingernails are long enough to ensure that only the nail comes in contact with the patient's skin, the fingernail serves as a good 'instrument'.

When one uses an instrument (or fingernail, used as such), the factor, able to affect colloidal equilibrium and used therepeutically, comes mainly into the category of physical factors — to some extent combined with the mechanical factor, friction. The back of the nail is, of course, used so that it glides lightly over the surface for supplementing action: also flat, but with much slower and heavier action, for draining or dispersing.

The same two factors (physical and mechanical) are applied when using the fingers, mainly the tips, for deep friction, pressure and manipulation. This technique is the one I most frequently use and prefer. But that is a personal choice. All are equally effective.

When there is an excess to be drained or dispersed, pressure is applied gradually, firmly, and increasingly gradually, until heavy pressure is reached. This is maintained until the operator feels a relaxation in the tissues. The pressure is then released very slowly, indeed almost imperceptibly. This represents a variant of what is known in osteopathy as 'inhibition'. The osteopathic practitioner sometimes uses the whole hand when a large muscle area is in spasm. Heavy pressure is maintained until relaxation of tension is felt, but the lift must be sufficiently gradual to ensure that a sudden lift does not have the effect of starting up the tension all over again.

For the supplementing movement, the fingers are applied rapidly to the desired depth and, as soon as the tissues respond (which will be felt as an increase in tension), pressure is quickly removed. Several applications may be needed before the tissues are felt to respond.

Percussion massage will be familiar to anyone who has studied the Japanese Kuatsu, or resuscitation, technique. It is not really a suitable technique for general use in one's clinical practice, but is admirably suited for emergencies. You should know something of the technique of percussion. This clearly is a mechanical factor. One, two, or three (very rarely more than three) short, sharp blows are given directly on the acupuncture point, using the end of the first phalange of index or middle finger. The fist is held closed, but with the operating finger having its first phalange in line with the metacarpal. The range of movement in delivering the percussive blow must not exceed four inches.

The heel of the hand is used percussively for an area such as the solar plexus: the knee for mid-dorsal vertebral points: toes for lowest vertebral points. I shall be mentioning several of the Kuatsu points when we come to consider the Govern Vessel meridian, in detail. These points would, of course, be suitable for techniques other than percussion.

While on the subject of mechanical factors, we should note that the Japanese have developed a highly effective use of Sound Waves — involving a peculiar sudden shout or cry, known as Kiai. The Kiai, using minor keys, flats, discords, produces syncope and paralysis by a nerve reaction which lowers arterial pressure, retards cardiac rhythm, and influences certain secretion reactions; whereas the Kiai in major key, sharps, and harmony of sufficient suddenness and intensity, induces excitation and acceleration of respiratory and cardiac function, etc.

Research into therapeutic use of ultrasonic frequencies at acupuncture points is being carried out; but I am not in a position to do more than merely mention the fact that research is being done.

7

The Five Elements, Continued

We continue to study the five elements and the doctrine of rhythm and changes in the energy polarities.

You will need to refer to the diagrams while you are reading this section. A simple set of diagrams and pictures should help make the notions clear. This is an important part of our study, and should be read and re-read until it is thoroughly understood. No analogy is perfect — but for our present purpose the analogy I shall use seems suitable, as far as it goes.

Imagine a motor-way or track of certain length, with a hairpin bend at either end (see diagram). A motor car is imagined as running round and round the track, in the direction indicated, in our diagram, by the arrows. Between the points A & B, C & D (the straight runs) the car travels at a steady 60 miles an hour.

In order to negotiate the hairpin bends, i.e. to change direction, there comes a point where measures have to be taken to slow the car down, so that at X it smoothly changes direction to go towards the straight again.

To attain 60 m.p.h. (considered as its proper speed between C & D), measures have to be taken to accelerate in such a way as to reach the required speed with optimum economy and safety.

An experienced driver knows exactly when to change gear, apply the brakes, depress the accelerator, shift the centre of gravity, etc., etc. These various operations he will carry out at almost precisely the same spots each time he makes the circuit. He chooses landmarks by the side of the track to guide him in his timing of these operations (see diagram).

The driver could, and probably in his mind would, label the operation by the landmark associated with it. To simplify the 'labels', we can use the following names for the successive changes, or stages of change: in one direction we have *water, metal, earth, fire, wood;* and in the other direction we have *metal, water, wood, fire, earth.* It is at these points that changes are to be made; they are points at which the balance, or smoothness, of running can most effectively be either disturbed or, if already 'out of gear', re-established. Between points A & B, C & D no significant influence is envisaged as likely to affect direction changes.

Now, supposing the tyres have worn smooth, application of the brakes at, let us say, the Fire point will not have the full desired effect. A skid might tend to develop. Therefore, until such time as new tyres are fitted, here, at the Fire point, the track surface could be suitably sanded. At this point — and that point alone — would 'sanding the track' have the effect of restoring or maintaining the proper circuit rhythm.

Let us now leave this analogy.

I have drawn a rough diagrammatic representation of a human being standing with his arms above his head (see diagram). You will see that the paths of the twelve organ meridians form a circuit traversed continuously by the Vital Energy. The circuit is continuous — so it does not matter at what point we elect to begin our consideration of it. Some teachers consider the circuit to begin with is the Lung meridian, whereas others begin with the Heart meridian. Personally, I have become so accustomed to taking the Heart meridian first (using Roman numbers in preference to the meridian names) that I choose this way. This conforms to the great majority of European acupuncture schools, and, therefore, for the sake of consistency it is well to adhere to an already established convention. Remember,

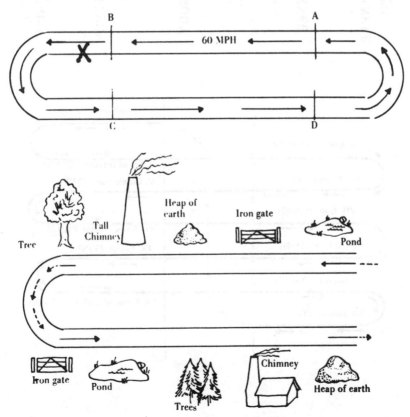

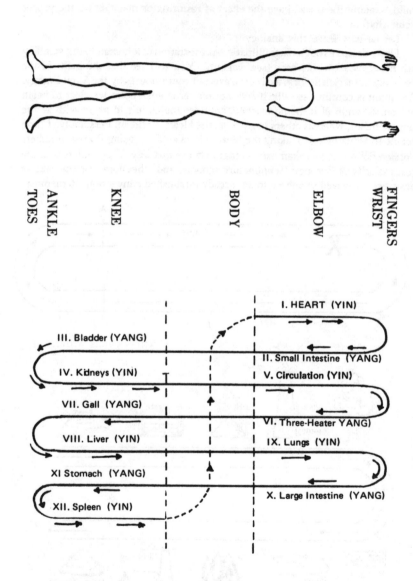

FINGERS
WRIST

ELBOW

BODY

KNEE

ANKLE
TOES

I. HEART (YIN)

III. Bladder (YANG)

II. Small Intestine (YANG)

IV. Kidneys (YIN)

V. Circulation (YIN)

VII. Gall (YANG)

VI. Three-Heater YANG)

VIII. Liver (YIN)

IX. Lungs (YIN)

XI Stomach (YANG)

X. Large Intestine (YANG)

XII. Spleen (YIN)

however, that this is a convention of convenience. In no way should it be looked upon as according greater importance to the meridian that happens to be mentioned first.

The Heart line (I) begins on the thorax, travels along the upper limb to finger-tips carrying Yin predominance energy. At the finger-tips the polarity changes and becomes characterized as Yang predominance energy. It now travels along the small intestine line (II) to the head, and from the head the Yang predominance energy travels on the Bladder line (III) to the feet. At the feet the polarity changes from Yang to Yin. From the feet the Yin predominance energy follows the Kidneys (IV) line to the thorax, and then, still Yin, follows the Circulation line (V) to the finger-tips. Once again, a change of polarity occurs. And so the circuit proceeds. At the extremities of the upper and lower limbs the polarity of the vital energy undergoes a change. In the central area, head and thorax, though the energy passes from one meridian to another, there is no polarity change (or, by analogy, 'no hairpin bend').

What we can get from this diagram, our rough schematic outline, is a visual representation symbolizing the fact that rhythmic changes of polarity predominance take place. The changes occur at the extremities (analogous to the hairpin bends at either end of the motor track).

The Energy Polarity predominance changes are most easily influenced at certain points near the extremities. These points, known as the Elements Command points, are labelled with the name of one or the other of the Five Elements. It will be noted that all these points are located at or distal to, the elbow, and at, or distal to, the knee.

In order to simplify the diagram I have reduced to minimum size the centre portion of the track, since, in these command points, we concern ourselves solely with the sections elbow to fingers and knee to toes.

There are some command points other than elements points within these same areas. These will be explained, in due course.

Have a look now at the Basic Five Elements Diagram — which we had in the previous lesson but which is given again in this lesson. I need to emphasize that, although each organ, or organ function, is classified as a Fire organ, Earth organ, etc., that is to say, characterized by, or associated with a particular related element, each "Element" (or whatever 'element' symbolizes) is not wholly one element, but only predominantly so. Each contains within itself something of all the others. This means to say, for example, that the Metal organs (lungs and large intestine) are linked with the Water, Wood, Fire, and Earth organs through the traces of these within the Metal.

I can illustrate this for you in another way. Each season of the year is linked to, and is, in some way, dependent upon, all the preceding seasons; and each also in some way influences to some degree all the seasons which follow.

Next year's harvest is inevitably tied up not only with this year's harvest (for upon seeds obtained this year will Spring sowing and then harvest next year depend — no seeds, no sowing; no sowing, no harvest) but, also, we see that Winter storage influences the Spring sowing. The fruits of this year will have been influenced by all the long succession of seasons coming before. We could go back-

The Basic Elements

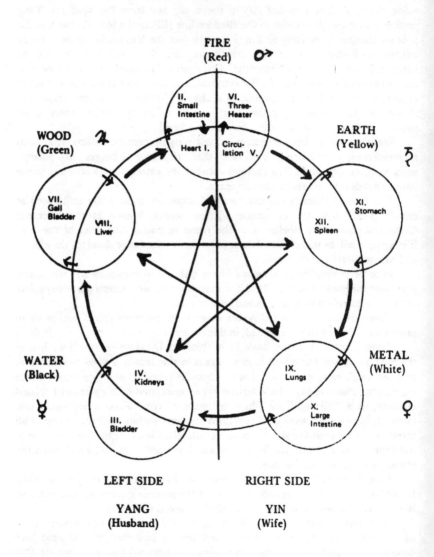

wards or forward in time more or less indefinitely, but, beyond a certain point, it is irrelevant to do so.

Balance and Imbalance

In perfect health there is a dynamic balancing of the 'elements' in quantity, quality and proportion.

"Perfect health" is, however, a concept that has no real existence; it is not a static condition; it is a process involving rhythmic creations of tensions and their relaxations.

It may sound somewhat of a contradiction: nevertheless, we say that a proper dynamic balancing is made up of rhythmically occurring imbalances and re-balancings to create the next dynamic imbalances. In a 'perfectly healthy' person there will always be found some relative imbalance. Somewhere, there will be an excess, and somewhere a deficiency, but provided these excesses and deficiencies happen at the proper times, in the proper circumstances, and within certain limits, they are not pathological but indicate health.

For example, it would be absurd to say that a perfectly healthy person is never hungry. Hunger amounts to an awareness or feeling resulting from a temporary excess of gastric juices relative to the temporary deficiency of aliments upon which to work. In health, hunger and satisfaction occur in proper rhythm.

Thus, excesses and deficiencies within certain limits, in proper relationship to one another, to time, to internal and external conditions, and so on, are counted as proper balances. We shall return to this when we consider what is known as the Chinese Clock, or times of the day when certain organs are more active; appropriate hours at, or between, which the activity or functioning of each particular organ can be most effectively influenced. Also, just as there are day and night rhythms of activity, so, too, there are seasonal, yearly, and other rhythms.

When excesses and deficiencies are what they should be and therefore do not come into the category of pathological imbalances, we refer to them, to avoid confusion, as normal balances. In the ordinary way, it is only when the excesses or deficiencies are such as to require treatment that we say there is an excess or a deficiency. I hope this is clear to you.

We now come to the question, how does the practitioner assess the state of balance of the Five Elements, or the state of the organ or function associated with each element?

If an excess or deficiency is great enough and/or has gone on for long enough, there will be externalized signs or symptoms of some sort or another. But, as I indicated in an earlier lesson, Chinese medicine has as its goal the detection of potentially pathological imbalances before the situation deteriorates and manifests as gross external symptoms. Then, having detected imbalance, the aim is to restore, by appropriate action, the proper balance and rhythm.

The diagnostic method characteristic of Chinese medicine is the pulses method. As you have already learned, the pulses enable one to know the state of the inner organs and functions, the state of the associated energy flow, and so on.

We now turn our attention to the Basic Five Elements Diagram in order to build up a logical pictorial link with the pulses and elements.

The basic diagram symbolizes for us a whole host of related items and factors. The arrangement of the elements in this order has its logic.

It illustrates the sequence from minimum (bottom left-hand corner of the diagram) rising through birth & growth to maximum or maturity (at the top of the diagram), then the falling-away through decrease or withdrawal, through balance to emptiness (minimum).

The organs associated with the elements are these:

YIN		ELEMENT	YANG	
Spleen	XII	Earth	Stomach	XI
Lungs	IX	Metal	Large Intestine	X
Kidneys	IV	Water	Bladder	III
Liver	VIII	Wood	Gall Bladder	VII
Heart	I	Fire	Small Intestine	II
Circulation	V	Fire	Three-Heater	VI

You will note that in our diagram a large circle, uniting all the elements, also divides each small circle into two. Inside the large circle are represented the organs that function continuously. These are the organs which store and distribute energy: whereas outside the large circle are shown the organs with an intermittent function and are concerned with feeding and excreting. If you refer back to page 24, you will recall this classification. The vertical line in our diagram, running through the centre of the Fire element, divides the diagram into a left hand and a right hand half.

The left hand and the right hand halves of the diagram coincide with the left hand and the right hand pulses. The superficial pulses are represented outside the large circle, and the deep pulses are represented inside the circle. I have drawn a separate diagram to show this even more clearly (see page 83).

The left hand/right hand relationship is known in acupuncture as the husband/wife relationship. In theory, the husband rules the wife. But there is a proper relationship of strengths of these two, and as long as this proper relative strength is maintained there is order in the household.

If the head of the house is weak (relative to the wife), there is disorder in the household. Excessive dominance of the husband over the wife results in tyranny, also in unbalance.

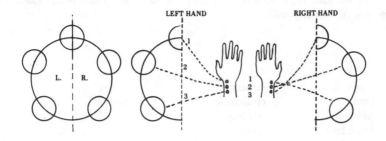

LEFT HAND   RIGHT HAND

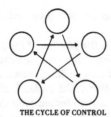

THE CYCLE OF CONTROL

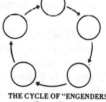

THE CYCLE OF "ENGENDERS"
(Generation Cycle)

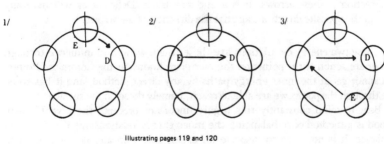

1/   2/   3/

Illustrating pages 119 and 120

4/   5/   6/

D = deficiency   E = excess

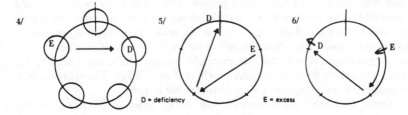

The left hand/right hand relationship, if unbalanced, results in the following sequence of "endangers":

Heart	endangers	Lungs
Liver	endangers	Spleen
Kidneys	endanger	Circulation
Small Intestine	endangers	Large Intestine
Gall Bladder	endangers	Stomach
Bladder	endangers	Three-heater

It does not take much reflection to appreciate the quite ordinary common sense of this.

The next item on the chart for us to note is the position of the arrows. There are two sets of arrows. The set of arrows going from one element to the next immediately following it forms a circulation of energy flow, known as 'the Cycle of Generation', and it is known as the mother/child cycle. Each element is considered as being the child (or engendered) of the element preceding; and it is also considered as the mother of the element following. This flow of energy is to be looked upon as indicating an energy flow between the organs themselves, not between the meridians. In this Five Element method we are dealing with deep internal (not the superficial external energy of the meridians) energy. The arrows indicate the direction of flow of energy. This is to say that excess always flows in the direction of these arrows. It is a one way track. Deficiencies will naturally travel in the opposite direction, against the direction of the arrows.

These two energy circulations are those which we aim to influence through appropriate action at the points on the meridians known as the Command Points. We cannot get at the inner energy paths by any direct method, and it has to be done through the points we are able to reach, namely those on the surface.

Bear in mind constantly this highly important precept: the Five Element method is a method of re-balancing the inner energy relationships if there is an unbalance. It is not used to disperse an excess into thin air, nor is it used to supplement an inner deficiency from outside. The method now being described represents a technique of re-balancing; therefore, it is only used when there is an excess on one or more of the organs and at the same time a deficiency on one or more of the organs. The whole essence of the method is one of transfer — a re-balancing of what is already there. In principle, balance is to be restored by taking energy from where there is a surplus to where there is a lack. We neither add to nor reduce the total energy, but we re-balance what is there.

Quite obviously, circumstances can occur when re-balancing of the elements, inter se, will not apply. Let us consider one such circumstance.

Suppose there is a general all-round deficiency of all elements, the question of re-balance by transfer cannot arise. This situation might well arise in a case of general weakness, let us say, after an operation or a long illness. The proper or normal energy quantum will have to be built up by other means. The action in such a case might be in the nature of a general tonic for the whole system, or by a careful conservation of the remaining energy allowing time for the quantum to be re-gained. One might not use needles, moxa, or massage, at all, but look instead to diet, rest and 'sunshine' methods.

In our enthusiasm for acupuncture as a needle technique, we should not be forgetful of other natural, and at times more expedient and efficient, ways of achieving what we want to achieve in the case.

Excess and Deficiency

Let us suppose that only one element is out of balance; not out of balance in relation to another element, but only with regard to the organs of that element. Taking an instance, let us suppose an excess on the liver, VIII, and a deficiency on the gall bladder, VII. It is obvious that re-balancing is required, not between different elements, but within the element itself.

In order to apply the rule of transfer from where there is more to where there is less and, of course, bearing in mind the 'waste not' rule, we would use the passage point on the meridian of the deficient organ; the polarity of treatment would be supply. One always acts on the meridian of the organ showing a deficiency, and acts by supplementing, or supplying. This is an instance of the the proper use of the passage points. As we shall see later on the passage points will also be used when we are re-balancing between different elements. The fact to be noted here is that the passage points are used to draw energy across the large circle. That is to say, either from an organ 'inside the circle' to one 'outside the circle', related in element, or from an organ 'outside the circle' to an organ 'inside the circle'.

Never forget this important rule: whenever you are applying the Five Element method always take supplementing action on the meridian with the deficiency, whether the deficiency has occurred of itself or has been artificially created by you.

Study the basic diagram until you have a clear and indelible picture in your mind, particularly of the direction indicated by the arrows. Surplus energy travels only in the direction indicated by the arrows.

I am now going to take several instances of occurrence of excesses and deficiencies to illustrate the principle of transfer or re-balancing. The examples I shall take are simple, but you will realize that it does not often happen that the cases are as simple as these. This does not matter, for once you have thoroughly grasped the simple you will be able to solve the more complex without over much difficulty. In all these examples, you should refer to the diagrams to get a clear mental picture of the procedure. The actual meridian point numbers I shall not be giving, but I shall refer to the points merely by their element names. See outline diagrams on lower part of page 83.

1. DEFICIENCY on XII (Spleen)   EARTH organ
   EXCESS on I (Heart)   FIRE organ

The use of the Generation Cycle is indicated here. Balance would be restored by drawing the Excess Energy from I (Heart) to XII (Spleen). The pathway is opened or unlocked by supplementing action at the Fire point on the Spleen meridian.

2. DEFICIENCY on XII (Spleen)   EARTH organ
   EXCESS on VII (Liver)   WOOD organ

The natural path for the transfer of energy is along the control cycle. Therefore, transfer is effected by supplementing action at the wood point on the spleen meridian. This draws the surplus energy along the pathway indicated by the arrow.

Always the energy must be drawn from where there is more to where there is less, along the natural paths in the direction indicated by the arrows, using either the generation or the control cycles or both cycles. For instance:-

3. DEFICIENCY on XII (Spleen)   EARTH organ
   EXCESS on IX (Lungs)   METAL organ

In this case, there is no single direct path along which to draw, and, as we can only draw along natural paths in the direction of the arrows, we have to use an intermediary.

First, we draw upon Wood by the control cycle by supplementing at the Wood point of the spleen meridian. This starts an energy movement by drawing on the normal towards the deficiency — thus creating a small deficiency on the Wood organ VIII (Liver). We now can act upon this artificially created deficiency to draw the surplus from the Metal by supplementing at the metal point on the liver meridian. This treatment involves action at two points.

In this case, you will see that energy could be drawn along other combinations of routes, using either three points, or four points. Refer to the diagram for the possible routes. In practice, we would not use any of the alternatives involving more than the two points, because the general principle of economy also applies to the number of points used.

      In the three examples I have just given, you will notice that these represent instances of imbalance among the Yin or storage-distribution organs; and the re-balancing is by the most economical use of the generation and control cycles. As an exercise, you should now take a pencil and paper and work out the ways and means of dealing with deficiencies on each of the other organs, IX, IV, VIII, I and V, and the excesses on each element, in turn. Do this thoroughly as regards the organs inside the circle, and make sure you have thoroughly grasped the principle before you pass on to the next part of this section.

If the deficiency is outside the circle and the excess is inside the circle, or vice versa, or both excess and deficiency are outside the circle, we have to apply the rule that: -

Internal/external and/or external/external imbalances cannot be balanced by the external organs alone. The passage channels must be used by acting at the passage points to draw the energy across the line.

As before, the most direct paths are to be preferred. I give several examples-

4. DEFICIENCY on XII (Spleen)   EARTH organ
   EXCESS on VII (Gall)   WOOD organ

First, act at the Wood point on the spleen meridian. Then act at the passage point on the liver meridian (see pages 51 and 52).

5. DEFICIENCY on II (Small Intestine)   FIRE organ
   EXCESS on XI (Stomach)   EARTH organ

Both of these are 'outside the circle'. The most direct path is shown by the arrows in the diagram. The points then would be acted upon in this order: -

The passage point on the small intestine meridian, The water point on the heart meridian, the earth point on the kidney meridian, the passage point on the spleen meridian (see pages 51 and 52).

6. DEFICIENCY on VII (Gall)
   EXCESS on XI (Stomach)

Act on points in this order : VII Passage Point,
VIII metal point, IX earth point, XII passage point.

Following the principles just described, take a number of instances of excesses and deficiencies and work out for yourself the most economical and direct paths.

The Moxa Technique

In the next lesson, I shall be continuing with the Five Elements. You will have had enough already for one dose. I must now go on to the next technique — Moxa.

All the command points may be massaged, and all except seven may be treated by moxa. See Table of Command Points on page 102.

The word, moxa, is simply the anglicized form of the Japanese 'mo ku su'', meaning "burning herb''. The traditional moxa is the dried leaf of Artemesia (common name, Mugwort). A small cone of dried artemesia is placed on the acupuncture point, and is lighted at the apex. It is allowed to burn down until the heat becomes no longer bearable—it is then quickly taken off before a burn is made causing a scar which might take a long time to heal.

I suggest that you, as the student, first apply a moxa to yourself, in order that you may experience it; it will then give you first-hand knowledge of the right moment to remove a moxa. I once made a scar on myself which took six weeks to heal — I would like you to do without that sort of experience.

Many different ways of applying heat to an acupuncture point have been tried over the centuries; but, up to the present, nothing has been found to equal the effectiveness of the traditional Artemesia. It is supposed that there may well be some actual curative property in the herb itself, quite apart from the heat generated — but this has not been measured, and it seems rather doubtful whether it is possible to measure such property at all.

The moxa technique is always used as a form of supplementing, toning or Yang polarity treatment except where forbidden.

Do not light the moxa cone with a match: use an incense or 'joss-stick'. This mention of joss-sticks brings us to an alternative way of applying Moxa. This is an attenuated way whereby all risk of burns and scars is reduced to a minimum. Since joss-sticks are, themselves, made with artemesia as the 'burning' factor, they may be used to treat the points. The method is to approximate the glowing tip to the acupuncture point until a 'sting' is felt. Withdraw it at once, and apply again. Repeat several times.

The massage techniques described in the previous lesson and the Moxa techniques have certain advantages over the needle techniques; the most obvious is that risk of infection is practically non-existent with massage and Moxa, whereas an imperfectly sterilized needle can have very serious consequences to both patient and practitioner.

In this course, I shall not go into details of the special moxa technique of the "heated needle": you should, however, be aware that such a technique exists. It is a special rheumatism technique, which may be used at certain special points only, and it involves inserting the needle into the proper depth and then heating the handle by means of the moxa wrapped round the handle — or heating by other means until the metal is glowing red hot.

The ordinary use of the moxa is highly effective, and many practitioners tend to use it in preference to the needle wherever this is possible. Some points are more suitable for moxa than for other methods — but watch carefully that you remember the points forbidden to moxa (some are obvious, some are not; they must, therefore, be memorized).

Small cones, "the size of a grain of rice", would be used, for example, at the finger- and toe-nail points; whereas points on the back, abdomen, and thorax would need cones the size of a hazel nut. It is up to each practitioner to use his own judgment and common sense over this.

Although in this course we have not yet studied the conception meridian, it is appropriate to mention now that there is one point on the conception that needs a special moxa technique. The eighth point on the conception meridian (.8) is in the centre of the navel. This point is forbidden to the needle, and may only be treated with moxa after filling the umbilicus with salt. We shall be referring to this point later in the course when we study the conception meridian, the governor meridian and the bladder meridian, where moxa would be the technique of choice.

It is wise, before applying a moxa, to make sure that the skin in the area is, in fact, sensitive. Unless this is done, a burn may be caused without the patient's being aware of it.

There is yet another reason for avoiding the causing of a burn, with a resultant scar. Scar tissue destroys the point: this means to say, scar tissue is a non-conductor of vital energy.

It is useful to remember this about scar tissue, for there can only be very few people walking about who have no scars at all. If a scar occurs on the path of a meridian, the path is diverted and a blockage in the meridian flow could be caused. This gives us a very sound reason why, in all cases of injury where scars are formed, the scar should be reduced by massage, as early and as thoroughly as possible.

Several clinical instances of long-term effect of injury have come to my notice. For example, a broken ankle, and the scar tissue, not reduced by massage, brought about several months after the accident various disturbances in the organs whose meridians were affected by the injury. One case in particular, I recall: these long-term repercussions showed as nausea, pruritis of the inner canthus of the eyes, headaches, lacrimation, intercostal pains, etc. The patient did not link these symptoms with a broken ankle! Nevertheless, these symptoms disappeared after the meridian paths around the ankle had been appropriately massaged and freed.

8

Application of the Five Element Laws

You will come across problems in the course of your clinical work. I shall give you some general advice on solving. Consider: (a) If the pulses show: Excess on VI (Three-heater) and on V (Circulation), Deficiency on IX (Lungs) and on X (Large Intestine) — what single point would you treat and why? (b) Excess is on all five organs, but no deficiency anywhere: where would you create a deficiency to draw off the excess?

I do wish to impress upon you that our aim is to teach you principles to be applied, and to make sure that you do thoroughly understand these principles. Only on this basis can you hope to become a good acupuncteur. If you rely only upon looking up a formula in a book, or looking up in repertories, you will never get beyond being a second-rate practitioner. So let me repeat: learn the Five Element laws, for these represent the basis of acupuncture therapy; never treat a patient without first reading the pulses. Do not be put off by anything you may read anywhere else, nor by anything anyone else may tell you, be guided by the pulses reading, whatever the symptoms may be.

The first problem showed the pulses pattern thus:-

Excess on both the Three-heater (VI) and the Circulation (V),

i.e. two of the Fire organs, and

Deficiency on the Lungs (IX) and Large Intestine (X), the two Metal organs.

We are asked for a single point at which treatment could logically be tried, with a good chance of success.

The first thing that appears to me is this: both Fire organs of the pair VI and V (three-heater and circulation) show an excess; therefore, it is possible that the passage points linking these meridians are not obstructed and might not need action. The same reasoning applies to the meridians IX and X (lungs and large intestine), the paired metal organs. If it be a case where the passage points are not obstructed, it would clearly suffice to take supplementing action on one of the meridians showing deficiency; the other deficiency would then of itself become replenished through an already unobstructed passage point.

This now leaves us with a choice between the Fire point on the lung meridian, or the Fire point on the large intestine meridian. How do we decide which of these to select? You might be guided by the symptoms in order to decide in your own mind which require attention most — shortage of breath, for example, in which case you would supplement at the Fire point of the lungs, or torpidity of the colon, when you would supplement at the Fire point of the large intestine.

If you are going to treat by either massage or needle, it would not matter which of these you selected to treat, but, if you wished to use moxa, you would have to choose to act at the Fire point on the large intestine meridian because, as you will see from the Table of Points on page 140, the Fire point on the lung meridian is one of the points forbidden to moxa.

I had a case very similar to this — the difference being that an excess showed on three out of the four fire organs. This was in a case of measles — the temperature was rather too high to be allowed to stay up that much, breathing was rapid and shallow, and the bowels were sluggish. By this I mean that, though the bowels were mechanically full and congested, the large intestine was deficient in energy. In this instance, because there was an energy deficiency on the large intestine meridian and, at the same time, the actual physical organ, itself, was affected, I used X.4, the point known as 'the organ or source point of the large intestine' (I shall explain the organ points in a moment). My patient was a child, and children do not seem to care for needles all that much, so I used massage. One can make quite a game of this massage with children — and it is as effective as any other technique. As soon as the massage was over, I read the pulses again: they showed improved energy balance, and this improvement indicated on the pulses showed itself outwardly by a bowel movement within about half an hour, and the temperature fell a whole degree within the hour.

In this case, I could have chosen the fire point on the large intestine meridian (X.5), using massage, moxa or needle. Probably with just as good results, perhaps even better, who knows?

Now, for our second problem. The pulses showed excess on all four fire organs, but no deficiency was revealed by the pulses. With the situation as it stands it does not appear to be a problem of re-balancing the energies within, for there is no deficiency into which the surplus can be drawn; therefore, we have to create one.

If you now turn to the Basic Five Element diagram and look carefully at the arrows indicating the natural pathways for the energy to flow, you will see that energy flows from the fire element to the earth element along the generation cycle pathway; so, if we can create a deficiency on the earth, the excess will tend to flow along the natural pathway to supply the deficiency. Thus, a short fast will create a deficiency on the stomach (meridian XI). There is also a natural pathway along the control cycle from fire to metal. A deficiency could be created in the metal by emptying the large intestine — how about a laxative? This gives us quite a good example of the logic of ensuring the bowels are kept open, and withholding food in cases of fever.

When occasion necessitates, deficiencies can be created in the other elements by similar procedures. A short fast will create a deficiency on the earth element, a long fast will create a deficiency on the fire element (small intestine). Emptying the bladder, or giving a diuretic, will create a deficiency on the water element; reduction of fats in the diet will create a deficiency on the wood element, etc.

This has now brought us to the subject of diet, and in the next section we turn our attention to the diet aspect of the Five Elements. Acupuncture is not all needles, but is much more far-reaching in its scope.

The Elements and Diet

The matter of diet is clearly of very great, therapeutic significance; for where is the sense of using a needle to re-balance energies if a faulty diet is allowed to continue, thereby re-creating the selfsame imbalance?

According to the Nei Ching, each Element creates a particular Flavour, which enters a particular organ, strengthens and nourishes a particular organ, is proper food for a particular organ. Each flavour has a special power, influence or effect; each flavour (if in excess) is counteracted by its own special counteractor, and counteracts an excess of a different one. This will be best appreciated if we set it out in tabular form:-

ELE-MENT	WOOD	FIRE	EARTH	METAL	WATER
create the flavours,	Sour,	Bitter,	Sweet,	Hot, Pungent, Aromatic,	Salty,
which enter the	Liver	Heart	Spleen	Lungs	Kidneys
and are the proper · food for the	Heart	Lungs	Liver	Kidneys	Spleen
The power of the Flavours are	Astringent Gathering	Drying Strengthen-ing	Harmoniz-ing Retard-ing	Dispers-ing	Soften-ing
An excess in the diet of is counter-acted by	Sour,	Bitter,	Sweet,	Pungent,	Salty
and counter-acts	Pungent,	Salty,	Sour,	Bitter	Sweet,
	Sweet,	Pungent,	Salty,	Sour,	Bitter.

PROPER FOOD RELATIONSHIPS

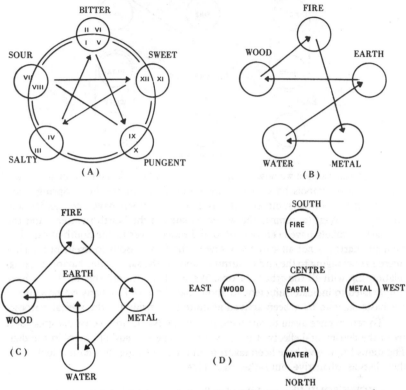

(A)

(B)

(C)

(D)

YELLOW RIVER MAP OF FU HSI (Adapted from the I CHING)
The earth in the centre signifies the soil, the earth substance, as distinguished
from the Earth as a heavenly body.

Using the basic Five Element diagram, which is repeated in diagram A above, you can follow the above sequences. If you do this, you will notice that the "proper food" relationships do not, at first sight, seem to follow a logical sequence.

The basic Five Element diagram we use today, and especially in this study, is not the only form in which the Five Elements have been represented in the past. According to the particular purpose of the symbol, so has the shape of the symbol undergone modifications.

In some arrangements of the symbol, the Earth Element, which is not associated with one of the points of the compass but with the earth centre, is placed in the centre of the diagram. In another arrangement, you will see that the earth has been split in two: one portion placed in the North-East, between water and wood, the other portion in the South-West, between fire and metal. You will also see that the wood element, and the metal element, have been represented split.

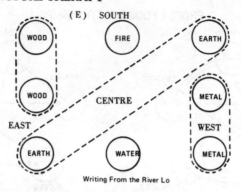

Writing From the River Lo

The basic diagram we now use may quite easily be deduced from diagram (e): the two wood symbols have been joined and placed in the East (Spring), fire remains in the South (summer), the two metal symbols have been joined and placed in the West (autumn), the water remains in the North (winter), and the two earth symbols have been re-united and moved over to the South-West. The element, Earth, is not allocated any one of the four seasons to itself, but is considered as belonging to the end of summer and, at the same time, having a special relationship with all the other seasons. We need not go into this further. I have simply tried to indicate sufficient to show that the Five Divisions we now use in our basic diagram have been arrived at quite reasonably for the special purpose.

To return once again to our flavours, in the Nei Ching we read a great deal about the detrimental effects of the flavours, if one exceeds all others in the diet. The items I now give have been taken from the Nei Ching, but do not look upon these lists as exhaustive, but rather as a guide.

EXCESS SOUR (that is, if the sour flavour exceeds all others
                        in the diet)

> Toughens the flesh,
> Is injurious to the muscles,
> The flesh hardens and wrinkles,
> The lips become slack,
> Causes the liver to produce excess saliva,
> And the force of the spleen will be cut short.

EXCESS BITTER

> Causes spleen energy to become dry,
> And stomach energy becomes dense, congested;
> Withers the skin;
> Body hair falls out.

> WHEN there is a disease of the bones one
> should not eat too much bitter.

EXCESS SWEET

Causes aches in the bones;
Heart energy will be full,
Kidneys will be unbalanced,
Hair on the head will fall out.

EXCESS PUNGENT

Knots the muscles,
Muscles and pulses slacken,
The spirit will be injured;
Finger and toe nails wither and decay.

WHEN there is an illness of the respiratory
tract, do not use too much pungent food.

EXCESS SALTY

The great bones become weary,
Muscles and flesh become deficient,
The mind becomes despondent

(In depression cases cut common salt
out of the diet)
Hardens the pulse,
Tears appear,
Complexion changes.
WHEN there is a disease of the blood,
do not use too much salty food.

Now let us have a few indications from the Nei Ching as to when to
prescribe, or use, the various flavours. I have retained the quaint terminology of
the Nei Ching.

SOUR

Sour food has an astringent or gathering effect; thus, the
heart suffering from tardiness means that it is devoid of
strength, and one should eat sour food which has an
astringent effect.
In connection with the liver, one uses sour food in order
to drain and expel.
Sick lungs have a tendency to close and to bind — eat sour
food in order to make them receive (gather) what is due to
them.
Use sour food to supplement and strengthen the lungs.

BITTER

When the spleen suffers from moisture, one should eat
bitter food which has a drying effect.

When the lungs suffer obstruction of the upper respiratory tract, eat bitter food which will disperse the obstruction and restore the flow.
One uses bitter food to drain the spleen.

SWEET

When the liver suffers from an acute attack, it indicates that there is an excessive fulness of the liver; one should quickly eat sweet food to calm it down.
One uses sweet food in order to drain and dispel in connection with the heart.

A sick spleen has the tendency to work tardily and laxily; then one should eat sweet food to set it at ease, i.e. supplement and strengthen it.

PUNGENT

Use pungent food to drain the lungs and make them expel.
When the kidneys suffer from dryness, eat pungent food which will moisten them.
Pungent food opens the pores and will bring about free circulation of saliva and fluid secretions.
If the liver has the tendency to disintegrate, eat pungent food to supplement the liver function and to stop leaks.

SALTY

Eat salty food to make the heart pliable (N.B. sea salt and not common salt), and to supplement and strengthen the heart.
Eat salty food to drain the kidneys and make them expel. (A far better method than "drinking pint after pint of water to flush them!")

Scanty as these notes may be, they do give us a start. It is well worth your while to realize that it is legitimate, sound 'acupuncture' to prescribe the diet in accordance with the pulse readings.

Consideration of the Five Elements is by no means exhausted. Each element, as you already know is traditionally associated with a colour. These colours were not chosen by the ancients arbitrarily, according to decorative whim or fancy! It is not difficult to see a connection between green and gall or bile. A bilious complexion is green. Lung under-activity is associated with pallor (white). Black rings under the eyes are associated with kidneys, etc. Colours of skin areas, organs, secretions, excretions, exudations, and so on, have, at times, valuable linkages giving clues to the meridians having energy imbalance.

Needle Techniques

If you think back to Chapter 6 where I offered an explanation of how acupuncture works and explained something about colloidal behaviour and the several factors able to influence colloidal equilibrium, you will already realize that the acupuncture needles represent simply factors able to do such influencing. Unless you have grasped the notions fairly well, you will be at a disadvantage in understanding the different needle techniques of the various schools of acupuncture and why, even though apparently contradictory, they all seem to work.

It is not necessary for us to worry ourselves over the pros & cons of the different schools' techniques; but we should be aware of some of their differences in teaching. In Europe, there is already growing up considerable dissension between what we may conveniently label ''the Gold and Silver Needle'' and the ''Steel Needle'' schools. Each claims the authority of antiquity in defence of its technique.

For the purposes of this study, we can consider the use of a 'needle' under four headings:-

1. One theory seems to revolve round the notion that the important factor is the fact of a puncture being made. In this case, it is considered of little or no importance as to what material the needle is made of, whether steel, gold, silver, metal alloy of one kind or another; even perhaps not metal at all. There was a time in history when thorns, bone or wood splinters, or sharp stones were used. That simple puncture is able to affect colloidal equilibrium is not scientifically disputed — indeed, it is recognized and placed among the list of ''mechanical factors.''

Soulie de Morant, who is looked upon by many as the source authority in Europe, writes that a simple dressmaker's sewing needle is often used, but usually with a head of some sort fitted to facilitate insertion and removal. When searching around for a readily obtainable needle, I have experimented with stainless steel sewing needles, surgeons' electrolysis needles, and others. In his book, Akupunktur als Neuraltherapie, Dr. Stiefvater tells about a colleague who became interested in acupuncture after having accidentally inserted a hypodermic needle into a patient without filling the syringe with anything. The effect on the patient was as if the intended fluid had actually been injected. This brought to his notice the fact that puncture could, in some instances, be at least as important as the injection of something! One practitioner of my acquaintance once told me that he considered it to be of little importance what he did at an acupuncture point; all he was concerned with was doing something at a correctly selected point.

2. There is the theory which attaches overriding importance to the material from which the needle is made, insisting that, according to whether the needle is of gold alloy or silver alloy (yellow or white metal), the effect differs.

Relatively short and rather thick gold and silver needles are used by followers of Dr. de la Fuye and others based upon Soulie de Morant. The thick needle is used on the authority of the statement made by Soulie de Morant that the thicker the needle the greater its efficacy, though, of course, the greater the thickness the greater the pain.

In an attempt to explain why these different metals bring about different polarities of treatment, Dr. de la Fuye draws attention to the fact of difference in ionisation of these two metals. Although I have used gold and silver needles (apparently with good effect), I have now discontinued their use for two main reasons: -

(a) They are too painful, and I am of the opinion that treatment should be as near painless as skill and art can achieve; and

(b) These needles are relatively soft, which means that the point not only soon becomes blunt, but, also, it may even be turned should the needle accidentally come against bone; it is then rather like trying to extract a fish hook from the unhappy victim.

Whether one agrees or not with the gold and silver theory, clinical results appear to indicate their therapeutic validity. In this case, the factor able to effect colloidal balance is to be found somewhere among the 'physical factors'.

3. There is the needle theory which stresses the form of the needle as of greatest significance. The form which seems to approximate most closely to the ancient traditional Chinese needle is specified as fulfilling the following requirements: fine as a hair (thus reducing pain to the minimum, the puncture being almost imperceptible), flexible (reducing risk of breakage) stainless steel, with the haft made of thin copper wire wound around one-third of the needle's length, and not soldered to the steel. This form of needle makes use of the principle known in electronics as "the thermo-couple": use is made of the difference in potential between the steel and copper surfaces to generate a minute electrical current — the amount and direction of flow of the current depending upon the metals used for the particular couple.

The needles I now use, and recommend come direct from China and are usually about one inch long.

This pattern or form of needle is suitable for those who follow the "thermo-couple" idea, but they are also admirable for those who follow the next theory (which, incidentally, I favour).

4. Under this fourth heading we consider the theory which attaches major importance to neither fact of simple puncture, material, nor form, but places emphasis upon manipulation of the needle. Followers of this theory use, as a general rule, similar needles to those just described; but some practitioners use needles where the copper wire of the haft is soldered to the steel; this naturally discounts the "thermo-couple" possibilities. Any fine flexible stainless needle is considered suitable, the guiding factor being the ease and precision with which the manipulations can be carried out.

Careful and detailed instructions are to be found in the Nei Ching, and other classical works, with regard to insertion, withdrawal and manipulation of the needle. I shall give only the essential rules which I, myself, use, and which are widely acknowledged as adequate for efficient acupuncture therapy. There are special manipulative techniques for producing special effects and for hastening certain processes, but their consideration is beyond the scope of this course, and

Needle Technique

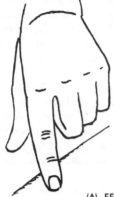

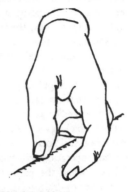

(A) FEELING THE POINT

(B) UNCOVERING THE POINT
AND READY TO PLACE THE NEEDLE

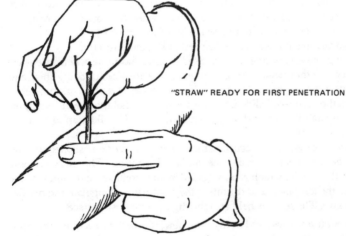

"STRAW" READY FOR FIRST PENETRATION

(C) NEEDLE IN POSITION, GUIDED BY THE
FINGERS OF THE LEFT HAND AND RO-
TATED (MANIPULATED) BETWEEN THE
THUMB AND FIRST FINGER OF THE
RIGHT HAND.

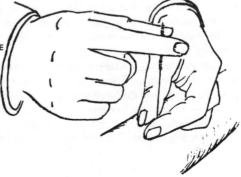

you do not need to know them. The essential rules must be faithfully observed. The point to be treated must, of course, be quite clearly indicated and accurately located. In some areas, there is practically no allowable margin of error — either you are on the point or you are not on it — ''nearly there'' is just not good enough. In other areas, there is some room for 'leeway'. In other words, we find that in some places the ''bull's eye'' is no larger than a pin-head, whereas in other places the ''bull's eye'' may be as much as three-sixteenths of an inch in diameter.

In order to supplement (tonify, stimulate, supply, etc.), the needle must be inserted when the breath has been fully exhaled, and to the required depth without rotating the needle: as soon as it is at the required depth, rotate the needle slowly until the flesh clings to the needle, then almost immediately quickly withdraw the needle while still rotating it. Close the hole by rubbing it firmly with the finger. The whole operation will take scarcely more than thirty seconds. The needle is withdrawn when the patient is breathing in.

In order to drain (disperse, calm, sedate, etc.), the needle is to be inserted rapidly, rotating it, during inspiration: and then left in position for at least ten minutes. It may have to be left in for half an hour, or even an hour. The time to withdraw the needle is when the flesh lets the needle go, or when it no longer clings to the needle. Withdraw the needle slowly, while the patient is breathing out, and leave the hole open; do not close the hole (do not rub it).

These two manipulations must be learned and followed strictly.

When using these very fine flexible needles, care has to be taken to ensure they do not bend — they need to be guided in. There are ways of doing this, and one is by using what we call a ''straw''. This is made of a thin, plastic tube, through which the needle will slide freely, yet which will hold the needle straight. The ''straw'' is slightly shorter than the actual needle. (The illustration on page 99 shows one in use).

The straw is placed on the acupuncture point; the needle is slipped in, and tapped with the forefinger to make the initial penetration. The straw is now quickly slid off the needle, which is now guided by the forefinger and thumb of the left hand while the forefinger and thumb of the right hand manipulate the needle, as described above. The straw is held at right angles to the flesh surface.

If you do not use a straw, and in my own view, it is better to acquire the habit of doing without a straw wherever possible, it is essential to have a way of ensuring that the needle is always placed exactly on the acupuncture point, which you will not be able to see while the thumb and forefinger are over the area. Refer to the illustration while reading the description, and you will find there is no difficulty at all.

Locate the acupuncture point to be treated by feeling for it with the left forefinger, so that the point is felt at the centre of the palmar surface of the last phalange. Now, roll the forefinger slightly to one side to uncover the point to be piqued. With the right forefinger and thumb hold the needle upright, the point not quite touching the actual spot to be piqued; the needle is held so that the end lightly rests against the left forefinger in contact with the place which a moment ago rested on the acupuncture point. If the left thumb is now moved into position (see illustrations), the needle will be firmly held between the thumb and forefinger of the left hand exactly above the acupuncture point. With the right thumb and forefinger hold the needle; press the needle in to make the puncture and to insert to the required depth. Then the needle is to be rotated by means of rolling the haft between thumb and forefinger of the right hand. The drawings should make this whole operation quite clear.

Before you try this out on a patient, practise it a number of times on a sausage, banana, orange, or whatever you may find handy for the purpose. Obviously, you will not be able to feel the "flesh cling" or the "letting go" until you pique actual flesh; but that part is not so important at the outset as it is to master the technique of getting the needle held in the right spot, and holding it with the left thumb and forefinger firmly enough to obviate bending or moving away from the point, and, at the same time, loosely enough to allow the needle to slide in as it is worked in with the right thumb and forefinger.

Remember you are manipulating Energy flowing in just subcutaneous pathways; only in very fleshy and muscular areas does the pathway go deep; therefore, do not insert too deeply. This injunction applies especially to the thorax, abdomen, head, face and neck. It is better to err on the side of making the pique too superficial than too deep. Do not puncture the arteries, and make quite sure that you do not pique a point forbidden to the needle.

Do not forget to sterilize the needles and to clean your own fingers (with surgical spirit or alcohol), and clean the patient's skin just around the acupuncture point you are about to treat.

Do not use the needle anywhere other than in an acupuncture point, and never in a swelling or tumour of any kind.

Use your "uncommon sense" and you are then unlikely to commit any foolish blunders or to have regrettable accidents. If you remember always it is a human being you are treating, you will proceed with loving caution.

The Points

In the next lesson, we shall be resuming the detailed study of the meridians, when you will gradually have the information given to you to enable you to find the points. In the meantime, learn the Table of Command Points.

You will notice, in the Table of Command Points, that the passage points are included; so, too, are the points known as the source or organ points. These are the acupuncture points which, according to tradition, have a direct link with the actual organ associated with the meridian. One uses these points either by themselves, or in association with other points on the meridian, if the organ itself is affected. You will notice that all the Yin meridians have their source point at the same site as their earth point. The Yang meridians have a special point for their source point.

All the element points may be either massaged or piqued ; but there are a few that are forbidden to moxa — note these carefully.

Command Points

ELEMENT POINTS, PASSAGE POINTS,
AND ORGAN (SOURCE) POINTS

Meridian	Wood Point	Fire Point	Earth Point	Metal Point	Water Point	Passage Point	Organ (Source) Point
(I) HEART	.9	.8	.7	.4	.3	.5	.7
(II) SMALL INTESTINE	.3	.5	.8	.1	.2	.7	.4
(III) BLADDER	.65	.60	.54 ▲	.67	.66	.58	.64
(IV) KIDNEYS	.1 †	.2	.3	.7	.10	.4	.3
(V) CIRCULATION	.9	.8	.7	.5	.3	.6	.7
(VI) THREE-HEATER	.3	.6	.10	.1	.2	.5	.4 ▲
(VII) GALL BLADDER	.41	.38	.34	.44	.43	.37	.40
(VIII) LIVER	.1	.2	.3	.4	.8	.5	.3
(IX) LUNGS	.11 ▲	.10 ▲	.9	.8 ▲	.5	.7	.9
(X) LARGE INTESTINE	.3	.5	.11	.1	.2	.6	.4
(XI) STOMACH	.43	.41	.36 *	.45	.44	.40	.42
(XII) SPLEEN	.1 ▲♦	.2 φ	.3	.5	.9 ▲	.4	.3

Part three

ORGAN MERIDIANS AND FACTORS OF TIME

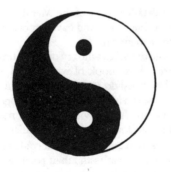

9

The Bladder Meridian (III)

We now resume our detailed study of the Meridian paths. Up to this point I have led you gradually into the work, and have not overburdened you with a vast amount of information to be memorized.

I know there are some teachers who try only to pump a lot of information in the students' heads, provide a 'book of words' and instructions, giving the student the idea that all he need do is collect the list of symptoms, look for the answer in his text book, insert a few needles — and hope for results! That is not the way we like to carry on. In my view, it is far more important that you understand, rather than that you memorize formulae.

There is, however, a certain amount of what could be looked upon as tedious committing to memory — for the paths and their points must be known. Set about this part of your study systematically and memorize, first of all, certain reference points which will then enable you to place those on either side and to consider the relationships of the different meridians. The meridians running from face to feet and from feet to thorax are not only long, but they also cross over each other and interlace here and there.

The Bladder Meridian (III) is the longest of these meridians, having in all sixty-seven points. It begins on the face and finishes at the little toe.

The points on the head will need very careful placing: I have presented enough charts showing these 'head points', so you should have no doubt whatsoever as to their exact location.

BLADDER MERIDIAN, III.

POINTS ON THE HEAD (Bilateral)

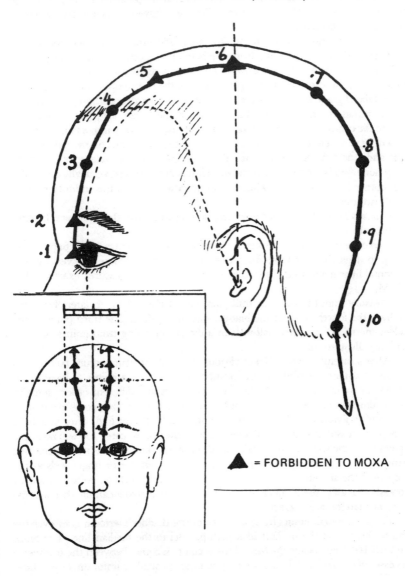

▲ = FORBIDDEN TO MOXA

The first two points on the bladder meridian are easy to locate. The first (III.1) is at the bottom of the small hollow at the inner corner of the eye: the second point (III.2) is above this at the inner end of the eyebrow, a slight depression there easily palpable. Both these points are forbidden to moxa, the needles are to be used with extreme caution, the pique being superficial only. I find, in practice, it is wiser to choose some alternative point rather than run any risks with a needle so close to the eye. Pressure, however, at the second point (III.2) is very effective.

For the remaining points on the skull we need to mark our reference points.

First mark the median line from the base of the occiput to the glabella (the point midway between the eyebrows). This line is divided into 14 1/2 A.U.M. Three of these divisions above the glabella mark the centre of the horizontal hair-line (maybe slightly above or below the hair-line, a lot depending upon whether the patient has any hair!) From this mid-, hair-line, reference point draw a line down to the centre of the external auditory meatus. This very important reference line will be your reference line (in later lessons) to place points on the gall bladder (VII) and stomach (XI) meridians. You will find that this reference line runs nearly horizontally along the hairline until it reaches the point vertically above the outer corner of the eye, from where it curves down towards the auditory meatus (see illustration).

It is assumed the subject is facing you squarely (or that you are looking straight into a mirror).

Now take the vertical line which passes through the centre of the pupil of the eye up to meet the hair-line: from this junction point (where the vertical and horizontal lines meet) to the midpoint of the hair-line, it measures exactly 1 1/2 A.U.M.

Measure from the hair-line mid-point one of these A.U.M. laterally: there you have the fourth point of the bladder meridian (III.4). The third point of the bladder meridian is exactly half-way in a direct line going from points two and four. See illustration.

After a careful examination of various charts of the acupuncture points, and consulting authorities of the exact location of acupuncture points, I have found that not all are in agreement. Some place the points in a different order; some in slightly different places; but one should remember that no two people are exactly alike, and individual differences are thus inevitable. If you find, after you have made your measurements and calculations with the utmost care, you feel no slight depression at the spot you have calculated, but you do find one a little to one side or the other (up to an eighth of an inch away), take what your finger feels as the true site of the acupuncture point. If you are unable to feel the point (hollow or depression) at all in the immediate vicinity of the calculated location, then assume your calculations are correct.

From the fourth point (III.4) the path of the Bladder meridian goes over the head to the base of the occiput in a path parallel to the median line. The tenth point (III.10) is just below the base of the occiput: it comes between the transverse processes of C.1 and C.2. It is quite easy to locate; usually painful under pressure.

To locate the sixth point (III.6), draw a line from the external auditory

BLADDER MERIDIAN, III

POINTS ON THE THIGH AND THE LEG

RIGHT LIMB ONLY IS SHOWN

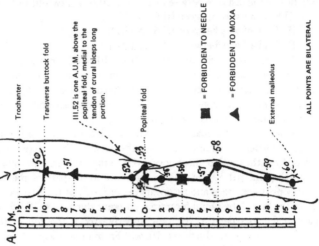

III.52 is one A.U.M. above the popliteal fold, medial to the tendon of crural biceps long portion.

Trochanter

Transverse buttock fold

Popliteal fold

External malleolus

■ = FORBIDDEN TO NEEDLE

▲ = FORBIDDEN TO MOXA

ALL POINTS ARE BILATERAL

A.U.M.

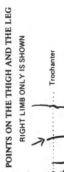

BLADDER MERIDIAN, III.

POINTS ON THE BACK

— III.38 SPECIAL POINT FOR ALL CHRONIC MALADIES

--- III.45 SPECIAL POINT FOR ALL CHRONIC AFFECTIONS OF INTERNAL ORGANS

Scapula

APEX

MEDIAN LINE

Spinous processes

Sacro-coccygeal articulation

Tip of Coccyx

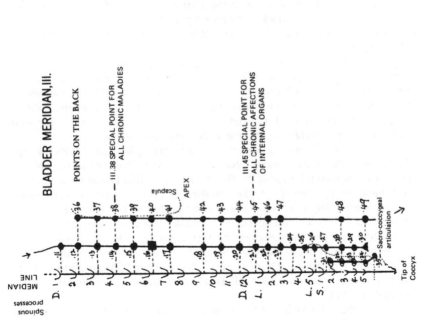

meatus vertically up and over the head to the other ear. Where this line crosses the path of the Bladder meridian is the sixth point (III.6). Point number five (III.5) is two-fifth of the distance between III.4 and III.6, i.e. two-fifths from .4.

III.8 is half-way between III.6 and III.10

III.7 is half-way between III.6 and III.8

III.9 is half-way between III.8 and III.10

Note that points five and six (III.5 and III.6) are forbidden to moxa.

Follow these detailed instructions with care, and place the first ten points on the Bladder meridian, referring to my charts and feeling for them on your own head (and/or on someone else's head) before you pass on to the study of the next group of points on this meridian.

Referring to the charts, you will see that the path of the Bladder meridian makes a bilateral double track down the back, with a triple track at the sacrum. Thus, from the tenth point it goes close to the spine in a straight line down to the thirtieth point (III.30) on a level with the lower part of the sacrum; here the energy path goes deep and reappears superficially at the first sacral foramen to go down the line of the sacral foraminae to point thirty-five (III.35) where the energy path again goes deep to reappear superficially at the top of the vertical inner scapular line at point thirty-six (III.36). From here it again goes straight down to point forty-nine (III.49), which is at the horizontal level of III.30. The meridian path then goes over the buttock to the fiftieth point III.50.

We shall now locate points eleven to forty-nine (III.11 to III.49). This is done by ''squaring''.

Our *vertical* reference lines are these: the median line, running down the centre of the spinous processes of the vertebrae; then a line, parallel to the median line, touching the inner border of the scapula (this we call 'the scapular line'); and another vertical line runs exactly half-way between the median and scapular lines. This line we call the 'paravertebral line'. The last, almost vertical line is on the sacrum; it passes through the centres of the sacral foraminae.

The *horizontal* reference lines are made by taking horizontal lines through the spaces between the spinous processes, just under the tips of the spinous processes. The eleventh point of the Bladder meridian (III.11) is at the level of the tip of the spinous process of D.1 (the first dorsal or thoracic vertebra). I remember using this point very effectively on a patient who had broken her wrist and after three weeks the fracture had not begun to mend. Massage at this point seemed to bring about an immediate response, for the patient said she felt something happening in her wrist. From that moment, the fracture began to unite, and mended very quickly. According to Dr. de la Fuye, this point is a ''Master Point'' for the bony structure of the whole body. (III.10 and III.11 act as a powerful tonic for the internal organs.)

In my chart, I have labelled each spinous process D.1., D.2., D.3., etc., for the dorsal or thoracic vertebrae, and L.1., L.2., etc., for the lumbar vertebrae. In order that there shall be no ambiguity or misunderstanding, whenever we refer to these horizontal reference lines I name the spinous processes both above and below the reference line, thus: point number eleven (III.11) is on the paravertebral line at the level of D.1/D.2, which means that the horizontal reference line is between these two spinous processes, but close to the upper one (or just below its tip).

The points on the paravertebral line are very important, as you will see in the next section of this lesson. You must be able to locate them precisely.

There is no need for me to describe the location of each point. I will, however, draw your attention to one or two aids to memory.

It will help you to place and memorize the first group of seven points if you note that:

III.11	is at the level	D.1/D.2
III.12		D.2/D.3
III.13		D.3/D.4
III.14		D.4/D.5
III.15		D.5/D.6
III.16		D.6/D.7
III.17		D.7/D.8

Point number sixteen is forbidden to the needle. You should be able to locate this point (III.16) and those either side of it, so as to be quite sure of avoiding accidents. If you feel for the lower apex of the scapula on left and right and join these by a horizontal line, you will find that this just about coincides with the level of D8/D9, which is the space without a point. Locate III.11 and the scapulae apexes horizontal and divide into seven spaces: one of these spaces up locates III.17, two spaces up locates III.16 which is forbidden to the needle.

From III.18, at the level of D.9/D.10, the points follow one after the other regularly down to III.30, which point is forbidden to moxa. Points III.31 to III.34 are easy to remember:

III.31	first sacral foramen
III.32	second sacral foramen
III.33	third sacral foramen
III.34	fourth sacral foramen.

III.35 is at the external border of the coccyx on the level of the sacro-coccygeal articulation.

III.36 is at the top end of the vertical scapular line on the same horizontal level as III.12.

III.41 at the level of III.17, then the 'space without a point'.

Study the groupings from the chart.

From III.49, which is at the same horizontal level as III.30, the path of the Bladder meridian now goes down over the buttock and down the middle of the posterior aspect of the thigh.

The reference points for all the meridians of the leg are, as follows. The great trochanter and the popliteal crease or fold; this distance is taken as 13 A.U.M. (Some charts I have examined take the transverse buttock fold as the reference line, but I have found, after carefully making the calculations using the different numbering of A.U.M, it seems that one always arrives at the proper acupuncture point. To avoid confusion, I have, as far as possible in this course, followed the same authority as regards reference points.) If you get accustomed to the method you are now being taught, you can rely on its serving you well.

The popliteal fold and the malleoli are the reference points for the leg. From the popliteal fold to the internal malleolus is 15 A.U.M., and to the external malleolus 16 A.U.M.

III.50 is in the centre of the transverse buttock fold (see chart) and III.51 is three A.U.M. vertically below III.50. Both these points are forbidden to moxa.

The acupuncture point in the centre of the popliteal fold, III.54, is forbidden to moxa, and it is also one of the few points which not only may be allowed to bleed; it is sometimes caused to bleed. Its special use in this respect is in cases of vomiting and diarrhoea; drawing a few drops of blood.

The remaining points are sufficiently clearly shown on the charts, and further description should not be necessary. Memorize all these lower limb points, especially the Element, Passage and Source points.

III.54 Earth Point	III.58 Passage Point	III.60 Fire Point
III.64 Source Point	III.65 Wood Point	III.66 Water Point
	III.67 Metal Point	

Make a careful note that III.62 is forbidden to moxa and that III.56 is forbidden to the needle.

The Bladder Meridian Association Points

In the previous section it was pointed out that certain points on the paravertebral line have especial importance. These are known as the 'Bladder Meridian Association Points'.

Many thousands of years ago the Chinese knew that, when an illness has become chronic and an organ is affected, there is a repercussion on the Bladder function, whose meridian becomes thereby unbalanced. The sick organ, its energy, and its meridian can be most effectively treated at certain points on the path of the Bladder meridian. For example, chronic disorder of the large intestine may be treated on the Bladder meridian at III.25, which is the Bladder meridian point associated with the large intestine.

These association points are sometimes known as the 'Dorsal Element Points'. Thus, III.25 is a metal association point.

There are rules for using these Dorsal Element Points. You will need to know three rules or conditions that must be fulfilled when using the Five Element Method with the Element Association Points:

(i) the malady is chronic

(ii) no acute symptoms are present, and

(iii) the energy imbalace is between different elements. They are not used if the imbalance is in one element only, such as the imbalance in the metal point when there is excess on the large intestine and deficiency on the lungs.

All the association points may be treated by needle, moxa, or massage; they are, however, especially suited to treatment by moxa. The general Five Element Rule applies in that one must always treat the deficiency by supplementing.

You will notice that we have included in our list of Dorsal Points one that is not an Element Point, but is of such importance that it should be memorized with them, namely, III.17. This is known as 'the Diaphragm Point'.

The Diaphragm Point is used for a wide range of disturbances and maladies, e.g. endocarditis, pericarditis, palpitations, angina pains, heart weakened by infectious diseases, weak, irregular, tremulous pulses, dyspnoea, suffocation, cough, bronchitis, pleuritis, asthma constrictions, nausea, vomiting, gastritis, stomach ulcers, stomach cancer, strictures and constrictions of all kinds, oedema, internal haemorrhages, night sweats, fatigue in the limbs, mental depression, etc.

BLADDER MERIDIAN, III.

POINTS ON THE FOOT

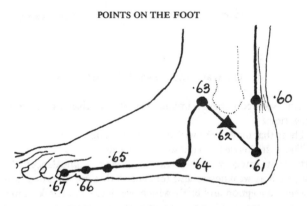

LEFT FOOT LATERAL ASPECT

NOTE: All points are bilateral, but only one side is shown.

Here is the list of the Dorsal (Bladder meridian) Element Points (Association points):-

BLADDER MERIDIAN ASSOCIATION POINT NUMBER	ASSOCIATED ELEMENT	ASSOCIATED ORGAN	POSITION ON THE PARAVERTEBRAL LINE; BETWEEN:
III.13	Metal	Lungs	D.3 / D.4
III.14	Fire	Circulation	D.4 / D.5
III.15	Fire	Heart	D.5 / D.6
III.18	Wood	Liver	D.9 / D.10
III.19	Wood	Gall	D.10 / D.11

III.20	Earth	Spleen	D.11 / D.12
III.21	Earth	Stomach	D.12 / L.1
III.22	Fire	Three-heater	L.1 / L.2
III.23	Water	Kidneys	L.2/L.3
˙ III.25	Metal	Large Intestine	L.4/L.5
III.27	Fire	Small Intestine	Level of 1st Sacral foramen
III.28	Water	Bladder	Level of 2nd Sacral foramen
III.17	Diaphragm Point		D.7 / D.8

NOTE: III.16 is forbidden to the needle; be careful when locating points III.15 and III.17.

Outward and Inward Disturbances

We can look upon energy imbalances or disturbances as coming into two main categories:
   (i) Those that move from within outwards, and
   (ii) Those that move from outside to inwards.

In the first category will come such energy imbalances that are constitutional, such as weaknesses and tendencies that are inherited, and those that arise between conception and birth which are not, so to speak, inherited from a long line of ancestors but are due to special circumstances connected with the expectant mother, her food, environmental conditions, what happened to her during pregnancy, and so on; what the birth circumstances and conditions were, when and where it took place, was it an easy or difficult birth, etc.

Other energy imbalances coming under this heading are those arising out of our own thinking and emotional patterns, feeding habits, etc.

Imbalances of this nature will show themselves in the pulses before they manifest in visible or detectable physical symptoms. An imbalance thus shown in the pulses without any external or overt symptoms is to be treated by the Five Element method. Energy re-balancing in this way prevents the imbalance from increasing and degenerating into outward distress. If one knows a constitutional weakness, it can be counteracted or compensated and ill health forestalled. This is the field of the Five Element method — the highest medicine — the prophylactic.

As far as possible I like to ascertain date, time, place and circumstances of every patient's birth. One usually has no difficulty in learning date and place, but time and circumstances are not always known to the patient. I shall have more to say about this when we come to the "energy tides" (daily, lunar, and seasonal).

Pulses may indicate imbalance and symptoms present. One, then, has to enquire in order to discover which came first — the symptom (outer disturbance) or the inner energy imbalance (the inner disturbance). Our aim is always to tackle the disturbance at its origin.

With regard to the second category, various factors coming from our environment may be the cause of a disturbance, as, for example, exposure to cold winds, heat, damp, injuries of numerous kinds, infections, excesses, etc. — these may create symptoms before the pulses are affected, and before the inner energy is disturbed. Sometimes, symptoms may reduce or even disappear; but when this disappearance is because they have worked their way inwards (perhaps through suppression by drugs) they cause serious inner imbalance which sooner or later will work its way to the outside again. A malady of this nature is chronic. If the chronic condition goes on for long enough, the inner disturbance will bring further symptoms to the surface and with them further deterioration, degeneration and ultimate terminal disease.

When the outward symptoms appear first, i.e. before the inner energy circulation becomes affected, it is quite in order to treat symptoms, for in this way we are treating at source; but, of course, the treatment is not suppressive. In other words, clearing up a superficial trouble before it has had time to go deep prevents it from reaching the inner energy at all.

Disturbances belonging to both categories can, and very frequently do, exist at the same time. We may have to deal with a superficial symptom first, in order to be able accurately to read the inner states. Obviously, if a patient is in great pain, one may have to tackle the pain first, at the least to calm the condition down.

In each and every case — *consider the patient — treat the patient — observe — reflect.* If you have not already done so, make up your mind here and now never to become a "formula monger", or what the ancients call "an inferior doctor, who does not treat patients but only diseases he had not the skill to prevent."

I will give one example of what, in my view, represented a legitimate symptomatic treatment. The patient had just had a tooth extracted, a local anaesthetic was given, the gums and surrounding tissues were just beginning to recover feeling; there was pain steadily spreading all over the face, forehead, and near the eyes, especially near the inner end of the eyebrows and over the top of the head. I considered two things needed doing:

First, deal with the pain and relieve it: second, but to me far more important, do something to speed up the elimination of the injected drug, before it had time to enter and cause disturbance to the inner organs, e.g. spleen and liver.

I hope you will follow this carefully, in order to appreciate the general line of reasoning. Once you really get down to doing your own thinking, you will not need to look up formulae in a textbook (nor memorize them); you will invent each time the correct formula for that special circumstance.

The dictum "drain for pain" clearly had to be applied. Pain always indicates an excess activity or excess energy accumulation at the site of pain. This energy required draining away from where it was in excess. One does not place needles in the centre of pain, but as close as one conveniently can, and always in an acupuncture point. Although in this course we have not yet studied the stomach meridian, it is expedient for me to tell you that the stomach meridian path goes over the face and lower jaw — the stomach meridian was affected by the tooth extraction and by the local injection. It was clear, therefore, that draining action was needed on the stomach meridian at points five and six.

Pain was also felt spreading at the inner corner of the eye and from there up and over the head — so, once more, it seemed clear that draining action was needed at the Bladder meridian points near the beginning of the Bladder meridian. For this I chose the third point (III.3). While the needles were still being inserted, the patient felt marked relief from the pain.

But the treatment was not finished. There were other things to be considered. There was no sign of an overall excess of energy or activity; therefore, this was not a case of dissipating excess energy into the air! But rather it was an instance of the need to draw the accumulation away from the painful area to some other area. The accumulation (or excess) was shifted to the other end of the Bladder meridian by supplementing action at Bladder point sixty-seven (III.67). This was done by moxa. At the same time, also by moxa, I took supplementing action at the large intestine source point (X.4), ''The Great Eliminator'', to stimulate the elimination of toxins from the system. Moxa treatment took but a few moments — the draining needles remained in situ for just over half an hour. The result was a complete, and very rapid, disappearance of all traces of pain and, as I estimated, vital energy had not been wasted but rather kept built up to cope effectively with what might otherwise have been a weakening situation.

Some acupuncture schools teach (and I have done so myself in the past when following a different teaching from that which I now follow) that draining and supplementing action should never be carried out at the same session on the same meridian. This may be reasonable enough where the points are close together, but when the points are at either end of a meridian, then the opposite polarity action has the effect of drawing a temporary excess away to another place without wasting it.

Remember this counsel always when draining. Do not deplete your patient. Whenever you drain, do so with caution, and as far as seems necessary select somewhere a suitable point on an appropriate meridian for supplementing action. This is in order to maintain a high level of energy reserves.

There are, naturally, occasions when simple draining action, per se, is all that is needed: but just be careful not to overdo it. The symptoms will undoubtedly disappear — but what sort of long-term trouble are you creating for your patient by reducing his energy reserves. I have even heard, for example, of a practitioner's inserting as many as forty needles in a patient at each of ten sessions! The symptoms were apparently slowly going — but so, too, was his vital energy! Within eighteen months (if not sooner) one might well expect the unfortunate patient to develop serious repercussions — and, very likely, no one would link the new malady with the acupuncture mishandling so long previously.

Use enough needles, or treat at sufficient number of points, to ''do the job'', but keep that 'enough' down to as few as are absolutely necessary.

KIDNEYS MERIDIAN, IV

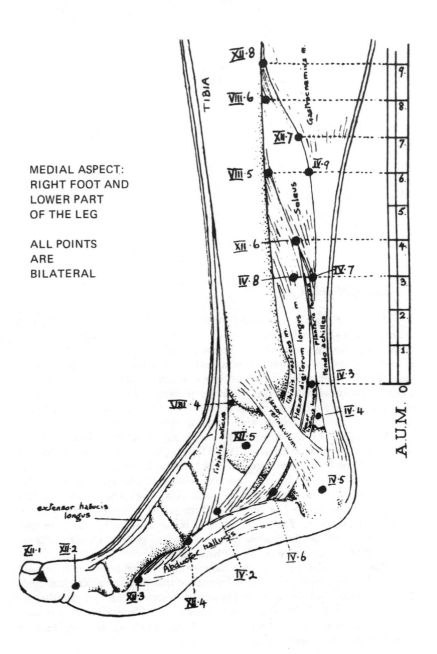

MEDIAL ASPECT:
RIGHT FOOT AND
LOWER PART
OF THE LEG

ALL POINTS
ARE
BILATERAL

10

The Kidney Meridian (IV)

Years after one has 'completed' the study of human anatomy (and passed exams), a person is often brought up with a jolt to discover just how 'rusty' that memory has become, even though one may daily be treating patients. I shall assume that refresher diagrams will be as useful to you as I find them to be to me. I have, therefore, taken considerable trouble to include in the charts for this lesson a much more detailed diagram of the lower section of the lower limb. Arteries, veins and nerves are not shown: in general, I find it easier to feel for tendons, ligaments or muscle crossings when locating Acupuncture points.

Although in this lesson we shall be studying the Kidney Meridian, IV, in detail, the points on both Liver (VIII) and Spleen (XII) meridians are included in the Chart, though I have not traced the paths of these last two.

A lot will depend, of course, upon the position in which the leg is held, and upon the degree of muscle tension, or relaxation, as to whether the Meridian paths will appear straight, or curved, and the points be more in line with one another, or otherwise. The actual mention of the muscles by name, or their tendons, together with the diagrammatic indication of location, should enable you to find all the acupuncture points without difficulty.

These three 'inside-the-leg' meridians are of very great importance, and will, no doubt, be frequently in use; it is imperative that they be known thoroughly. The Kidney meridian has many points for the treatment of sexual disorders and malfunctions — physiological and psychological. The Element points, naturally, are as necessary to know as on any other of the meridians, and they figure in several formulae for special uses.

It is necessary that I draw your attention again to the fact that authorities disagree with regard to the placing and numbering of several Kidney meridian points, especially on the lower part of the limb. *In addition to the acupuncture points on meridians, there are, on the foot [and round the ankles], no less than thirty-three acupuncture points that are not on any meridian path.* Is it then surprising that authorities disagree as to exactly how many of these points belong to a meridian, and which do not? What matters to us is that what we learn works. Learn one system first, and learn to use it. Later on, you may well be able to compare different teachings, and arrive at your own reasoned modification of one or another system. No one, in this world of ours, is in exclusive possession of all the right answers — therefore, it is best to remain ever flexible and open-minded.

The Kidney Meridian, IV, has its first point on the sole of the foot between two pads: one under the base of the big toe (metatarso-phalangeal articulation) and the other at the base of the metatarso-phalangeal articulations of the other four toes. I his first point (IV.1), though not expressly forbidden to the needle, should not be used unless circumstances absolutely require it, as it is just about the most painful of all points to pique. I well remember being present when a patient had a needle inserted at IV.1 — his scream haunted me for a long time.

Nevertheless, this point is very useful indeed, especially for massage action. It is a special point to use in all cases of emergency when there is retention of urine. Deep massage at this point brings about a good release. The point is massaged by placing one hand over the dorsum of the foot and, with the knuckle or distal end of the first phalange of the index finger of the other hand, working from the centre of the two pads towards the meridian second point. Massage always in the direction distal to proximal, or up the meridian path.

This same point (IV.1) may be effectively treated by deep firm pressure. I had an excellent instance of this on a patient whose main trouble was psychological, due to pent-up emotion, or repressed tears. This point is as useful to bring about an 'emotional release' as it is to release other fluid. About a minute after applying pressure with my thumbs at this point, the patient burst into tears and wept practically throughout the treatment session. The outcome was, however, extremely beneficial to the patient's whole organism. It is not for nothing that the ancient greek medical tradition declares that ''tears and laughter are two potent healers.''

The second point (IV.2) is just under the navicular (or scaphoid) prominence, or where the tendons of the tibialis anticus and tibialis posticus come to a V (see diagram). This is a useful point to bear in mind for sexual disfunctioning, e.g. insufficient sperm, orchitis, female sterility, dysmenorrhoea, uterine congestion and prolapse, vulvar pruritis, etc.

This Kidney meridian path now goes behind the ankle, just anterior to the Achilles tendon, at the horizontal level of the most prominent part of the internal malleolus (the subject standing in the anatomical position). The posterior tibial artery can be felt pulsating at this point (IV.3). Remember this point for dyspnoea and cough, diaphragm spasm, and various mouth and throat conditions.

The fourth point (IV.4) is vertically below the third point, and lies between the Achilles tendon and the tendon of the flexor hallucis longus (see diagram).

IV. KIDNEYS MERIDIAN

POINTS .1 to .10

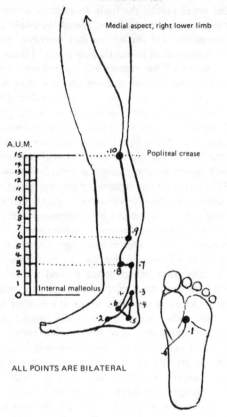

Medial aspect, right lower limb

A.U.M.

Popliteal crease

Internal malleolus

ALL POINTS ARE BILATERAL

(For a better view of points .2 - .9, see detail chart on page 164.)

Point Five, IV.5, is vertically below IV.4.

IV.6 is vertically below the internal malleolus. Some charts place it a lot nearer to the malleolus than we show it: they place it at the crossing of the flexor retinaculum and tibialis posticus tendon. We place it between the tendons of the flexor digitorum longus and the flexor halucis longus. It seems a pity to me that there should be dispute as to the location of this point — it is such a very important point, being the Control Point of one of the 'Extraordinary Vessels', the Yin accelerator — but the study of these Vessels goes beyond the scope of this Course.

The seventh point on the Kidney Meridian is known as one of the Very Great Points. I shall have more to say about this and other points on the Foot in the next Section of this Lesson. Referring to the Chart, you will see that our reference points are: the level of the popliteal crease and the level of the internal malleolus.

The distance between these two references is divided into fifteen A U M. IV.7 is 3 A U M proximal to the malleolus. IV.8 is about 1 A U M anterior to IV.7, and at the same horizontal level. IV.9 is three A U M proximal to IV.8.

IV.10 is just beyond the inner extremity of the popliteal crease (when the knee is in full flexion). This is the water point on the Kidney meridian, and will be in constant use when applying the Five Element method. IV.10 can be felt to lie behind the cracilis tendon and in front of the tendon of the semi-membranosus.

From the inner extremity of the knee-fold (popliteal crease) the path follows the line of the interstice between the semi-membranosus and semi-tendinosus to about half-way up the thigh; the path then curves over towards the lowest or medial extremity of the groin and goes over the pubic bone. At 1-1/2 A U M from the pubis symphysis is the eleventh point, IV.11, which is just above the upper border of the pubic bone. This is the only forbidden point on the Kidney Meridian: it is forbidden to the needle.

Our reference points for the lower abdomen are, starting from below to upwards, the upper border of the pubic bone and the centre of the umbilicus. The distance between the two is reckoned to be 5 A U M. From IV.11 the points are placed vertically one above the other parallel to the median line: thus, IV.12 is one A U M above the pubic bone; IV.13 is two A U M above the pubic bone, etc.: IV.16 is at the horizontal level of the umbilicus.

For the upper abdomen we take the umbilicus as our southernmost level; above the level of the lower end of the sternum. This distance measures 8 A U M.

IV.17 is two A U M above the level of the umbilicus; then points 18, 19, 20 and 21 are at one A U M intervals.

IV.21 is two A U M below the tip of the sternum, or one A U M below the tip of the zyphoid process.

The path of the Kidney meridian now turns slightly laterally to pass up and over the 7th and 6th ribs to the Fifth intercostal space; then vertically parallel to the median line, half-way between the median line and the nipple. IV.22 is in the 5th I.C.S., IV. 23 in the 4th I.C.S., IV.24 in the 3rd I.C.S, IV.25 in the 2nd I.C.S, IV.26 in the 1st I.C.S. and IV.27, the last point, is in the space between the 1st rib and the clavicle.

Points on the Kidney Meridian

If you remember your early gruelling in human anatomy (if not, refer to your own anatomy textbook), you will notice that the level of IV.19 (half-way between the umbilicus and the tip of the sternum) coincides with the Western anatomists' Transpyloric Line; and the level of IV.15 coincides with the Western anatomists' Transtubercular Plane.

On the thorax the Kidney meridian follows what is known in Western Anatomy as 'the Parasternal Line'.

In addition to studying the lessons of this text, you will get no end of useful information by carefully comparing the positions of the Chinese Acupuncture Points, Reference marks, Lines and Meridians with the actual underlying structures.

KIDNEYS MERIDIAN, IV

POINTS .11 to .27

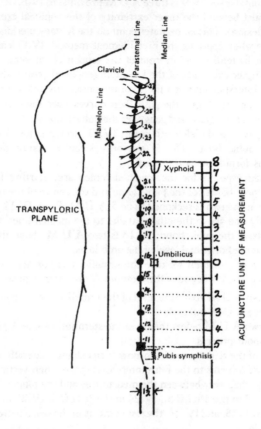

It will then come as no surprise to you to find that, for example, IV.18 is used in cases of Constipation — for the Transverse Colon passes directly under this point. IV.19 is indicated in vomiting, flatulence, icterus, eye congestion and misty vision; on the left side, IV.19, the transpyloric-line, underlying structures include the upper border of the transverse colon, the lower portion of the stomach, and, deep, the centre of the Left Kidney: while on the right, IV.19, the underlying structures include the Right Lobe of the Liver, the Duodenum (close to pylorus) and, deeper, the Right Kidney.

I have often marvelled at the genius of the Chinese masters of several thousand years ago, who devised a measurement technique for locating so accurately specific sites — whatever the patient's shape or size might be. In spite of the unlimited number of so many differently shaped individuals, certain relationships appear sufficiently constant as to enable one, with confidence, to apply the measurement standards and location rules of Acupuncture.

The sixth point, IV.6, has certain special uses. According to tradition, it has an especially powerful action upon the throat. In emergency, pressure quickly applied at this point might well save a human life. It is indicated, for example, in the case of a wasp, or bee, sting on the tongue or throat, when the part swells and there is danger of asphyxia. It is also an emergency point in concussion cases, or when there is unconsciousness but no convulsions, and blood oozes from the ears and mouth. I have used this point to relieve the distress arising from wasp, bee, gnat, or other insect bites anywhere on the body. There has always been rapid relief.

According to the Indian ''Tridosha'', there are Six Jewels, or six outstanding homoeopathic remedies. One of these is Sepia, which, in its potentized form, is administered for the same wide range of disorders that the Chinese Acupuncture Point, IV.7, is used. From your own understanding of the Five Elements you will realize that, since this point, IV.7, is the Metal point of the Kidney meridian, it would be used when the Kidney Pulse showed a deficiency and the Lung and/or Large Intestine Pulse an excess. Watch for the symptoms that go with just such a pulse combination.

IV.7 is also included in a well tried formula to control sweating, namely, IV.7 and X.4.

The long list of symptoms and conditions given by Dr. de la Fuye for which IV.7 is used includes: Renal atrophy, Acute renal hypofunction, Surrenal capsule insufficiency; Arterial hypotension; Cold feet, cold in the bones; Borborygma, abdominal tympanism; Excess salivation; Urethritis; Sacro-lumbar pains; Icterus; Paraplegia, paralysis of the feet, weakness in all four limbs after shock; weak eyes, misty vision; Continuous sweats in spite of feeling cold to the bone; Disorders arising out of intestinal worms; malaria, intermittent fevers; prolapse of urinary bladder, blenorrhagia; Dysphagia; Maladies of the spine marrow; Palpitations, etc., etc. This point should be considered in cases of bleeding haemorrhoids.

IV.10 will be of especial interest to practitioners who have much to do with athletes and their injuries. In order to strengthen weak knees, Moxa should be applied to IV.10; also, in cases of displaced, semi-lunar cartilege, or tendency to such displacement, use Moxa here. A glance at the Repertory will show you the use of this point in various genitalia disorders.

In the previous Section, I mentioned IV.3 as having special action for Cough, Dysnoea, and the like. It is used in conjunction with IX.10 (Lung point ten) as a general formula for Lung conditions where cough is a symptom.

You will appreciate how this could have effect when you note that IV.3 is the Earth point and Source point of the Kidney meridian. This would mean that Supplementing at this point would, (a) stimulate the kidneys themselves to more lively function and, (b) draw excess energy from the Earth Element (Stomach and Spleen). IX.10 is the Fire point on the Lungs, and would be used in Supplementing action to drain excess from the Fire organs to supplement deficiency on the Lungs.

11

If you are told that for a particular patient with bleeding piles, IV.7 is the indicated point — what pulses reading would you expect, and why — and what treatment would you consider suitable?

This first question should have presented no difficulty to you at all really; for, since IV.7 (the fourth point of the Kidney meridian) is the metal point of the Kidney meridian, and you know that when the Five Element method is applied one always acts upon the Deficiency, one would expect the Kidney meridian to show a Deficiency. The two Metal Organs are the Lung and Large Intestine: therefore supplementing (toning) action on the Kidney Metal point would draw upon the Metal Organs, and we would therefore expect either the Lung or the Large Intestine, or both, to show excess.

Since IV.7 is not one of the forbidden points, any technique could be used — massage, moxa, or needle to supply action. My own preference would be moxa — but that is a personal idiosyncrasy.

Let us suppose a patient comes to you six months after a severe fall on the left shoulder, dislocating the sterno-clavicular articulation and bruising the acromio-clavicular articulation area. He has come for treatment for boils on his face, close to his nostril and (for no reason) his jaws are swollen. He also suffers from excessive flatulence. All these symptoms, he says, have arisen since his accident from which he has 'quite recovered' except for some stiffness in his shoulder. His pulses show Deficiency on IV and X, but no excess. What treatment (up to five visits) would you suggest, and why?

The fact that the pulses show deficiencies and no excesses indicates that the Five Element Rule is not applicable here; because it is not simply a matter of re-balancing the energies. A re-balancing can be done only when there is somewhere an excess and somewhere a deficiency.

If a dislocation at the sterno-clavicular articulation has, in some way, injured the area of the last point of the Kidney meridian (IV.27), has severe bruising at the acromio-clavicular articulation will have, in some way, damaged the path of the Large Intestine meridian around its fifteenth and sixteenth points.

Thus, we conclude that the cause of the present condition is peripheral; and the disturbance in the Meridian Energy Flow has worked its way inwards (by the lapse of time) to affect the organs of those injured meridians. That the Large Intestine organ itself has been affected is evidenced by the present symptom — boils at one extremity of the Large Intestine meridian. Moreover, the path of the Kidney Meridian goes over the abdomen and a disturbed abdominal organ might well appear to affect the meridian energy path in the vicinity of the organ disturbance.

What one would do in this case is to massage not in tonification nor in sedation at acupuncture points; but massage with a view to breaking up any adhesions that might have accumulated in the injured area, and thereby free the peripheral energy pathways. It would be advisable, on the first visit, to palpate the entire length of the Kidney and Large Intestine Meridians; and by massage make sure that any adhesions, knottings, stiffnesses, lumps, and so on, are worked clear.

This procedure might well take up a great part of the second visit as well. On this second visit, which could be conveniently arranged for the next day (or day after), if the actual symptom on the last point of the Large Intestine Meridian has not shown signs of responding, one would pay particular attention to the actual organ itself by taking toning action at the first point (X.1) and at the organ point (X.4), the Great Eliminator.

Ensuring freedom of flow for the meridian energy of both Kidney and Large Intestine will assist the eliminatory function and tone the system up generally. The whole of the second visit would be well spent on massage to the paths of these two meridians and to the toning action at X.1 and X.4. Do not omit to read the pulses before and after treatment, and make a note of your findings. The treatment should show some immediate effect.

Dislocation at any articulation inevitably involves some .stretching of ligaments and/or damage to cartilagenous tissue and/or muscles. Cartilagenous and ligamentous tissue is dealt with by action upon the meridian associated with this kind of tissue — namely the Kidney Meridian which is associated with bones, cartilege, and ligaments. Local stimulation or supply action would be taken at the kidney point twenty-seven (IV.27) by using a moxa. You could, of course, use massage only.

At the third visit, if in your view the obstructed flow in the two meridians IV & X is now restored, you would be guided by the pulses indications and apply the Five Element Rule to bring about whatever re-balancing now appears needed. By this time it should show itself in the pulses — that is, of course, if any re-balancing at all is needed.

It would be an erroneous approach to the case if you set out, at the first visit, to treat the boils, swollen jaw, and flatulence symptoms by treatment at acupuncture points such as X.1, X.4, etc., or to treat local stiffness of the shoulder at X.11, while ignoring the massage at the site of the injury.

I have assumed here that three treatments would suffice; but it may be that even after five treatments the trouble has not completely cleared up, and it is not possible to give further treatments. You (and your patient) may rest assured that what you have done will have given the patient's system and tissues the best possible opportunity of spontaneously improving and correcting themselves — for you will have set free (or made more free) the natural healing energies in your patient.

Another problem: You are travelling by train with a middle-aged woman and her daughter. The mother suddenly finds it hard to breathe. Her face begins to cyanose, tongue swells, and there is soon severe distress. You realise that she will be a 'gonner' within three minutes unless immediate action is taken. What emergency acupuncture would be appropriate?

Tell the daughter to loosen the woman's clothing and remove her shoes. Keep the patient propped in a sitting position. Take hold of the patient's hands (one in each of yours) and press deeply and firmly at the ninth point of the Lung Meridian (IX.9) with the intention of stimulating lung action.

This point (IX.9) is known as 'the Corpse Reviver'; it is also poetically called 'Absorption of the Spirit of Good'. This is the organ point on the Lung meridian — toning action here stimulates oxygen absorption, and (as the Earth point of the Lung meridian) draws vital energy from the Earth organs to the Lungs.

By now the patient's shoes should be off. Let go of her right wrist and use your now free hand to dig into the sole of the foot at the first point of the Kidney meridian. Press hard and deep. This should bring about an immediate urination, which among other effects will have a positive influence on restoring or maintaining body temperature. This point, IV.1, is at the opposite end of the Kidney meridian to the possible location of the disturbance, namely, the lungs and respiratory tract. This point will stimulate heart action as well as relieve lung congestion and apnoea.

The Gall Meridian (VII): Points on the Head

The path of the Gall meridian, VII, will be considered in three groups of points. The first group comprising those on the head; the second group those points on the trunk; and the third group consisting of all the points on the lower limb.

The name of this meridian is shortened to Gall meridian, for not only is it more convenient to have a shorter name, but also this shorter form serves as a reminder that removal of the gall bladder does not mean the disappearance of the meridian. Surgery may impair the activity of the energy having the gall function, but it does not bring that function, in the wide sense of the term, to an end.

This meridian is of very great importance and needs careful study. Some of the points are difficult to place. The difficulty is not so much for the student as for the teacher; because the various texts and charts I have examined are either not sufficiently precise, or they do not all agree one with another. After having made a careful study of the underlying anatomical structures, and having used many of the points at the placings I give in this text, it seems to me to be sound to work

GALL BLADDER MERIDIAN, VII

HEAD POINTS OF MERIDIANS II, III, & VI ARE ALSO
SHOWN TO GIVE THE RELATIONSHIPS OF THEIR PATHS

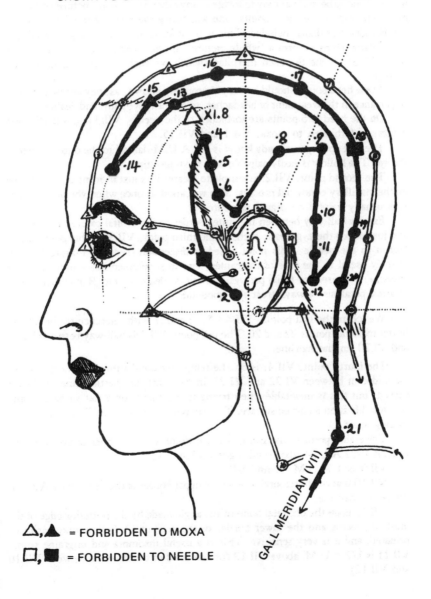

△,▲ = FORBIDDEN TO MOXA

□,■ = FORBIDDEN TO NEEDLE

with the acupuncture point placing as I have detailed them. Do not ever lose sight of the fact that various authorities disagree — and, one day, it may be your lot to re-place some points and give your reasons for modification of what is given to you here.

At first glance the head points seem to follow a complex zigzag pattern; but if they are carefully studied from the written descriptions and from the charts, they will be found to be quite as easy to locate as any other set of acupuncture points. In my detail chart of the 'head points' you will notice the paths of the Three-heater and Bladder meridians included. This is in order to facilitate study by enabling their relationships to form a 'whole picture'. In the chart I have also included a point (XI.8) on the Stomach meridian (which we shall be detailing in a later chapter).

These head points should be very thoroughly known, as they are of immense importance in the treatment of headaches, migraines, eye pains and deafness.

On the head two points are forbidden to the needle, VII.3 and VII.18: two points are forbidden to moxa, VII.1 and VII.15.

The first point you already know is 1/2 A.U.M. lateral to the outer corner of the eye. The hollow is easily palpable with the finger-tip.

The second point, VII.2, is simple to locate; it is just in front of the earlobe on the maxillary condyloid process. You will know at once when you are on it, as it is usually painful on digital pressure.

Exactly half-way between the outer border of the orbital cavity and the ear, and just under the zygomatic arch, is the third point, VII.3 — this point is forbidden to the needle. This point, used in dispersion (sedative massage) is extremely useful in the case of migraines; and in supplementing action (moxa or massage) it is used for facial paralysis, tinnitus, deafness, etc. Remember, when treating paralysis, always treat the good side.

We locate the gall points, VII.4, .5, .6 and .7 with reference to the Three-heater meridian points 22 and 20. The gall point. VII.7 is half-way between VI.22 and VI.20 on the hairline.

The fourth point, VII.4, is on the temporo-frontal suture, vertically above the midpoint between VI.22 and VI.23. In the chart the 'vertical line' is shown curved; but this is inevitable when trying to represent, on a flat surface, a line which in life is on a curved surface. The gall points, 4, 5, 6 and 7, are at an even spacing apart.

The eighth point of the gall is a Great Point for all manner of eye troubles, and it is 1 1/2 A.U.M. above and slightly behind VI.20.

VII.9 is 1 A.U.M. behind VII.8.

VII.10 is at the horizontal level of the upper border of the helix and 1 A.U.M. inside the hairline.

VII.12 is on the occipital bone in the angle made by the posterior edge of the mastoid process and the lower border of the occiput. A hollow may easily be palpated, and it is very sensitive. This is a useful insomnia and migraine point. VII.11 is 1/2 A.U.M. above VII.12 (or one-third of the distance between VII.10 and VII.12).

From the twelfth point the Path of the Gall meridian travels up and forward over the head to the forehead horizontal hairline. Where this line is intersected by a vertical line drawn from the outer end of the eyebrow (VI.23) is the eighth point on the Stomach meridian. This point is mentioned now because it is useful to illustrate the relationship of the row of hairline points.

The fifteenth point of the Gall meridian is on the hairline vertically above the centre of the pupil. The thirteenth point of the Gall meridian (VII.13) is half-way between the eighth Stomach point and VII.15.

VII.14 is vertically below VII.15, on the forehead, half-way between VII.15 and the centre of the pupil.

On several patients I have noticed a peculiar puckering of the skin at this site: all these patients, several years previously, had been operated upon for removal of this gall bladder.

From VII.15 the path runs parallel to the Bladder line over the top of the head to the nineteenth point, VII.19, which is at the same level as III.9.

VII.17 is 1/2 way between VII.15 and VII.19
VII.16 is 1/2 way between VII.15 and VII.17
VII.18 is 1/2 way between VII.17 and VII.19

The twentieth point (VII.20) vertically below VII.19 is under the occiput on the posterior of the neck at the horizontal level of the tip of the mastoid process.

VII.21 is at the base of the neck just anterior to the trapezius muscle, at the bottom of the hollow formed when the arm is raised.

You will recall (Lesson 5) that the fifteenth point on the Small Intestine meridian is on the trapezius muscle at the horizontal level of the spinous process of the seventh cervical vertebra. In cases of hiccups, stand behind the patient and, with your thumb, on II.15 and forefingers (or middle fingers) on VII.21, grip hard as 'pincers'. The sufferer will squirm, but the hiccups will go.

The Gall Meridian (VII): Points on the Torso

The diagram which I have prepared for this book has been drawn to as large a scale as the paper will take, in order to show the detail in such a way as to ensure perfect accuracy. Even on so large a scale drawing we still have the difficulty of representing on a flat surface a line that is curved in nature.

VII.22 lies in the axillary line in the fourth intercostal space; and VII.23 is one A.U.M. anterior to VII.22. Some authorities show the path from VII.21 to VII.22 as passing in front of the shoulder and some behind the shoulder. This discrepancy is not important as regards the placing of the points, but, of course, it does assume some significance when, for example, a patient has sustained an injury which, if it lay across the meridian path, could impair the flow of energy in some measure. As I have found it difficult to discover sound reasons for deciding one way or the other, I think we would be on the safe side (in such a case) to assume that the path runs both in front and behind. It would seem better to massage an injured area on the assumption that a meridian pathway has been

GALL MERIDIAN, VII

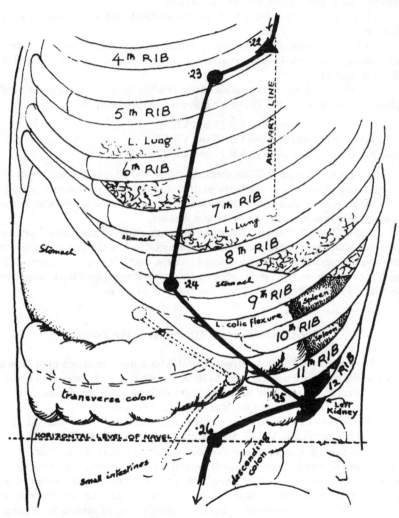

NOTE: All points are bilateral. Only one side shown.

affected, than to assume a pathway has not been affected and therefore not massage. Although in one case we might massage when it is not needed (but will certainly do no harm, probably do good) we avoid the possible error of omitting massage when it is needed.

VII.22 is forbidden to moxa.

Curiously, it seems to me, VII.23 has especial value when there is pain in swallowing and difficulty in speaking. On two occasions I have noticed patients with a pronounced stammer experience rather sharper pain at VII.23 than would ordinarily be expected. Both points VII.22 and VII.23 have value in local symptoms, such as intercostal neuralgia.

VII.24 is vertically below the nipple in the eighth intercostal space. This is a useful point for all stomach and liver disorders. We have used it clinically with success in hiatus hernia.

GALL MERIDIAN, VII

ALL POINTS BILATERAL

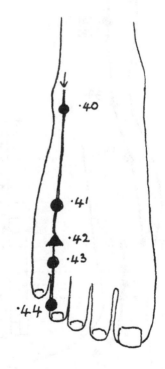

 = FORBIDDEN TO MOXA

GALL MERIDIAN, VII

RIGHT LOWER LIMB

ALL POINTS ARE BILATERAL

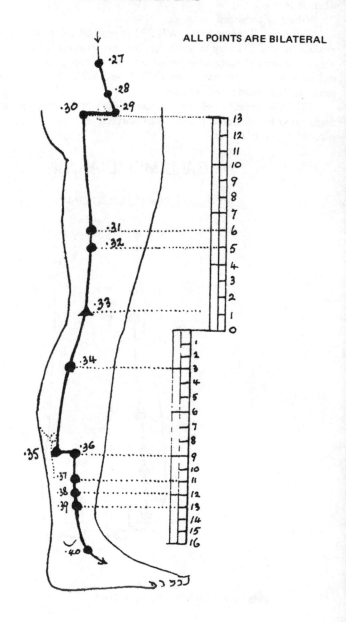

VII.25 lies just beyond the tip of the 12th rib. The proximity to the splenic flexure of the colon, the kidney and spleen on the left side; and to the liver, kidney, and hepatic flexure of the colon on the right side will clearly show this point would be indicated for such disorders as colic, flatus, nephritis, vomiting, and arterial hypertension.

VII.26 is found by 'squaring'. Draw a horizontal through the umbilicus and a vertical through the tip of the 11th rib. Where they cross is the twenty-sixth point. Three A.U.M. vertically below VII.26, on the hip, is VII.27. The small hollow is easily found, and under pressure pain will be felt shooting down the thigh. You will be in no doubt when you have found the point.

The next three points are also easy to find: VII.28 is one A.U.M. above the trochanter (firm pressure elicits considerable discomfort). VII.29 is just anterior to the most prominent part of the trochanter; and VII.30 is posterior to this same bony protuberance, in the middle of the deep hollow formed when standing erect and with muscles tensed.

VII.31 is 6 A.U.M. proximal to the popliteal fold.
VII.32 is 5 A.U.M. proximal to the popliteal fold.

VII.33, which is forbidden to moxa, will be felt in a slight hollow on the lateral aspect just proximal to the lower head of the femur (one A.U.M. above the politeal fold).

Like the Yin meridians of the leg, the Yang meridians of the leg cross and interweave somewhat. You should study the charts until you have formed (and are certain of retaining) a clear picture of the relative positions of the leg points.

VII.34 will be felt 3 A.U.M. distal to the popliteal fold, just under the head of the fibula. This is the Earth point on the Gall meridian. It is a Great Point. It is used in conjunction with X.11 as a general toning formula, to augment vitality and generally strengthen the body's powers of resistance.

When VII.34 is used in conjunction with VII.30 this combination acts powerfully on the whole of the lower part of the body.

VII.35 is one A.U.M. vertically below III.58, which is the same as saying that VII.35 is seven A.U.M. above the external melleolus. VII.36 is one A.U.M. horizontally anterior to VII.35.

VII.37, .38, .39 are respectively 5, 4, 3 A.U.M. above the external malleolus. You will notice, on looking through the repertory, that in addition to their use for local symptoms these points are also used for dealing with various symptoms occurring towards the other extremity of this meridian; e.g. VII.38 for axillary adenitis; VII.37 is also used for psychological disturbances of a "gall" nature.

On the foot itself, VII.40 is one A.U.M. anterior to and below the external malleolus. This point is traditionally linked directly with the organ itself and would be used alone or in conjunction with other points on the Gall meridian if the gall bladder itself was disturbed. The remaining points may easily be located from the charts. VII.42 is forbidden to moxa.

24 Hour Tidal Rhythm

You will remember from our first discussion on the Five Elements and the change of Polarity of the Energy, that the Energy flows continuously throughout the twenty-four hours through the meridians. There is no break in the continuity of flow, while there is life; though the flow may be disturbed — either too much flow or too little. We now have to introduce the rather important subject of the twenty-four hour Tidal Rhythm.

It is as if there were a tide, or crest of a wave, and this tide (or wave crest) takes two hours to pass through each meridian in turn. This two-hour period of optimum activity represents the best time for taking acupuncture action on the meridian concerned.

At the beginning of the two-hour period, when the tide is beginning to rise, is the best time for stimulation: one hour after this period when the peak has passed is the best time for calming, soothing, dispersing action. This sounds reasonable enough.

Twelve hours after (or before) the high tide begins the low tide occurs in the meridian. This low tide two-hour period is the time when the energy activity in the meridian is at its minimum.

The chart shows the 24-hour clock, with the meridians marked against the appropriate hours of optimum. The meridian point given in each case is known as the Horary Point. In other words, this is the point associated with the same Element as the Meridian, itself. For example VII.41 is the Wood point of the Gall meridian which is itself a Wood meridian.

The value of these Horary points is this: if the time of treating a particular meridian coincides with its two-hour optimum period, the point of choice upon which to take action will always be the Horary point: for, at that time, it would be the most effective point on that meridian.

You may have been able to spot another use for these Horary points (I hope you have). In the above example, let us suppose that according to the pulses there is no excess shown anywhere and the only deficiency shows on the fall; one would choose the Horary point and act upon it at (or soon after) 11 p.m. in stimulation.

Obviously the Horary points of the Liver, Lungs and Large Intestine would not often be used as Horary points — for who expects a patient to call between three o'clock in the morning and seven o'clock in the morning? Nevertheless, if you are a visiting practitioner, and are called out at night, you may well have occasion to use them — they should therefore be known.

While on the subject of VII.41, it should be noted that this is one of the Great Points of Acupuncture. It has been found to have marked therapeutic effect in skin diseases (Eczema, psoriasis, dermatitis, etc.) as well as having a special action on pains in general, but especially upon head pains and aches.

At this point, VII.41, one can very effectively bring about a good balance of the energies flowing through the six longest meridians, III, IV, VII, VIII, XI and XII. If VII.41 is coupled with VI.5 one has a powerful formula for dealing with all manner of pains, neuralgias and articular swellings. This coupling should be

THE 24 HOUR TIDE AND HORARY POINTS

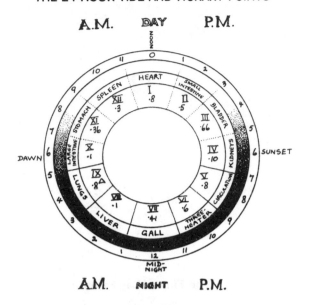

NOTE: IX .8 is the only Horary Point forbidden to moxa.

thought of in cases of general exhaustion, weakness and depletion after a long or serious illness. Traditionally, it is used to help rebuild the Energy resources.

Only one of the Horary points is forbidden to moxa; in all other cases any treatment method is permissible. The point forbidden to moxa is IX.8.

If you have been regularly reading your own pulses at hourly intervals during your waking time, you will have already noticed that the pulse strength in each meridian varies rhythmically. For example, between five and seven in the morning the Kidney pulse will be barely perceptible, yet twelve hours later this same pulse will be quite strong. That is as it should be, in proper accord with the kidneys' high and low tide. You would not look upon these readings as indicative of any pathological conditions, unless there were other signs as well.

This high and low tide is an important factor to be taken into account when reading the pulses. One needs to assess with care whether or not a pulse reading is as it should be. You will, of course, also consider whether an organ itself is full or empty. This last factor has to be weighed against the time of day. In our next lesson we shall be considering yet another pulse factor, namely the Seasonal Rhythm.

Pay special attention to the pulse in relation to the time of day, and make sure you have a clear picture in your mind of the Clock and Meridian times of Maximum and Minimum.

12

The Time of Day Factor

Let us question an instance of the Five Element Method.

In this instance, there is somewhere an excess and somewhere a deficiency. The surplus has to be transferred to where there is a lack. We naturally assume that the excess on the bladder may be greater than one might ordinarily expect: between the hours of three and five in the afternoon the pulse of the bladder would tend to be at its optimum anyway.

It is a general rule to use as few points as possible; thus, if one can effectively take short cuts, then one does. In this case then we would first try treating VII.43 in supplementing action. This point is the Water point of the Gall meridian, and it is possible that action here might well suffice to draw the excess off the bladder to the gall. As soon as the action has been taken the pulses are read. If the pulse indicates response no further action is needed. If, on the other hand, no response is shown by the pulse one would treat the points in this order: supplementing action at VII.37 (which is the passage point from the Liver meridian to the Gall); supplementing action at VIII.8 (which is the Water point of the Liver meridian); finally, supplementing action on the Kidney meridian passage point from the bladder (IV.4).

How do we take pain into account? One can use a formula, such as that given on page 132, VII.41 and VI.5. We would have to consider whether this formula could be applied in this case. One can use local points and draining action (Drain for Pain). The local points for draining action would be III.7, VII.1, VII.11 and VII.14. These points then would seem to be quite definitely indicated to relieve the pain, and we act on them. But since no excess is indicated on the pulses the energy which we are dispersing requires to be replaced somehow. This we would do by taking supplementing action, preferably by using moxa, at the opposite end of the Gall meridian, or very near the opposite end. The Three-heater, which shows the deficiency, needs supply action. These last two factors seem to point to VII.41 and VI.5, the formula mentioned above, in supplementing action (by use of moxa).

Each practitioner will have his own way of arriving at what he considers the appropriate points in every individual case. We should not, therefore, look upon any one answer as the only correct solution to a problem. The action I have given here simply represents a way in which I would reason for solving the problem.

It does not seem to me to be an instance where the Horary Point of the Bladder meridian would be appropriate, although it could be said that the energy which is being drained off at III.7 might be replaced by supply action at the opposite end of the Bladder meridian, and that the Horary Point would be chosen for this purpose (III.66).

I would certainly seriously consider the fact that a severe deficiency with no excess anywhere should be treated, in addition to any action at acupuncture points, by some attention to augmenting energy by suitable dietary changes. I would recommend the patient to increase the proportion of grain in his diet — the grain should be whole wheat; it would also be in order to advise reduction of the proportion of sweet foods, because sweet foods tend to have a draining action on the Fire organs.

The Liver Meridian (VIII)

The Liver meridian begins at the big toe, close to the ungual angle, from where it follows the outer dorsal border of the toe and first metatarsal. It then goes on the dorsum of the foot, over the tarsals, curving slightly medially to pass over the ankle's articulation anterior to the internal malleolus. It then ascends to the knee, following the internal edge of the tibia in a straight line to the lower edge of the head of the tibia; it then curves posteriorly to the knee; then forward curving; curving again to follow up the interstice between the rectus femoris and sartorius to the groin; then, following the border of the external oblique, it passes in front of the tip of the eleventh rib, along the costal border to its last point, which is where the mamelon line crosses the costal border (below the cartilege of the ninth rib).

I have included a detail sketch of the points on the internal aspect of the knee, in order to show the relationship and relative positions of the eighth Liver Point, the tenth Kidney Point and the ninth Spleen Point.

Although there are but 14 points on the Liver Meridian, all are of importance, and you will frequently find they are indicated in practice. The only forbidden point on the Liver Meridian is point number 12, which is in the groin; this point is forbidden to the needle.

VIII.1, the first point, is also the Wood point and Horary point of the Liver Meridian.

VIII.2, the Fire point of this meridian, is in the space between the first two toes, close to the big toe. Used in conjunction with the third point it is highly effective in the treatment of cramp occurring anywhere in smooth or striated muscles. You will find this combination of great usefulness in emergencies; not infrequently a patient has an attack of cramp when on the plinth. The effect is usually instantaneous. The third point is in the angle formed by the first and

LIVER MERIDIAN, VIII

POINTS .1 to .4

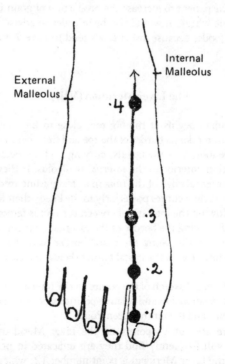

External Malleolus

Internal Malleolus

·4

·3

·2

·1

NOTE: All points are bilateral, but only one side is shown.

second metatarsals, this point being also the Earth and Organ (or Source) point of the Liver Meridian.

Some authorities do not mention the use of these points, VIII.2 and VIII.3, for cramps and spasms; but I have used them so often, with instantaneous relief, that I feel it would be a serious omission if I did not mention them.

The fourth point, VIII.4, the Metal point is one A.U.M. from the internal malleolus, anterior to this malleolus. The hollow can be readily palpated: firm, digital pressure here will usually elicit discomfort if not actual pain.

VIII.5 is six A.U.M. above the level of the internal malleolus. This point is

LIVER MERIDIAN, VIII

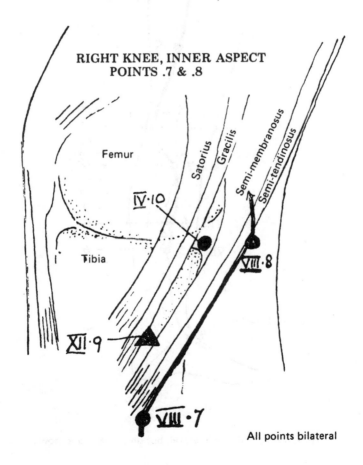

RIGHT KNEE, INNER ASPECT
POINTS .7 & .8

Femur

Satorius

Gracilis

Semi-membranosus

Semi-tendinosus

IV·10

Tibia

VIII·8

XII·9

VIII·7

All points bilateral

LIVER MERIDIAN, VIII

RIGHT LOWER LIMB
POINTS .4 -.9

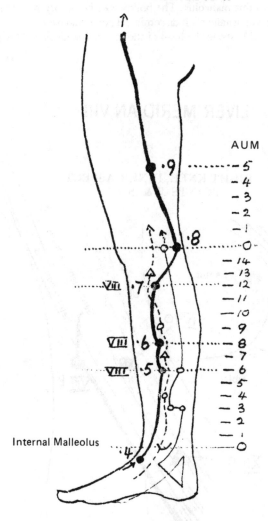

NOTE: All points are bilateral, but only one side is shown.

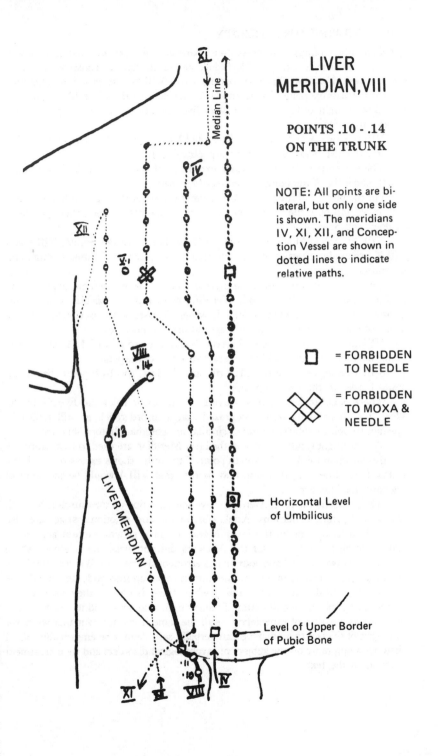

LIVER MERIDIAN, VIII

POINTS .10 - .14
ON THE TRUNK

NOTE: All points are bilateral, but only one side is shown. The meridians IV, XI, XII, and Conception Vessel are shown in dotted lines to indicate relative paths.

☐ = FORBIDDEN TO NEEDLE

✖ = FORBIDDEN TO MOXA & NEEDLE

— Horizontal Level of Umbilicus

Level of Upper Border of Pubic Bone

Median Line

XI

IV

XII

VI

VIII

LIVER MERIDIAN

.14

.13

.12

.11

.10

XI

II

VIII

IV

useful for either cramps or spasms and for paresis; but especially that of the lower abdomen and urinary bladder. Elderly folk sometimes have a 'constant drip' as a result of vesical paresis; this indicates the use of VIII.5 in stimulation. This fifth point is the passage point linking the Gall Meridian to the Liver Meridian, and should be thought of in connection with liver afflictions, such as hepatic colic, cholecystitis, etc.

VIII.6 is two A.U.M. above VIII.5; and VIII.7 is four A.U.M. above VIII.6 (or three A.U.M. below the level of the popliteal fold).

The eighth point is at the inner extremity of the popliteal fold (see detail chart), and is the Water point of the Liver Meridian.

For the placing of the points on the inner aspect of the leg, study the charts with care, and note the relative positions of the points on the other meridians (Kidney and Spleen).

VIII.9 is 5 A.U.M. above the popliteal fold. These last two points, VIII.8 and VIII.9, are used in cases of anuria, and locally for spasm in the medial thigh and leg muscles.

The next three points are close together. VIII.10 is on the femoral artery one A.U.M. below the groin. Dr. Wu Wei Ping gives this as a special point for inducing sweats or sleep. They should, however, be used with discrimination on a male patient on account of their "aphrodisiac" tendencies.

VIII.11 is also on the femoral artery, but in the groin. VIII.12 is also in the groin, lateral to .11, two A.U.M. lateral to the root of the penis.

VIII.13 is at the tip of the 11th rib, and the last, the 14th point, below the costal border in the mamelon line.

There is an ancient Chinese saying, "The Liver rules the Eyes." In the West, too, it has long been recognized that a disordered liver will reflect in eyesight troubles — blurred vision, scintillating scotoma, photophobia, etc.

As one might expect, points on the Liver Meridian are used to treat jaundice. For this affection think of the fourth point. If the pulse shows excess on the Lung and/or Large Intestine, then you may be sure that VIII.4 would be the point of selection for jaundice.

The points on the Liver Meridian have special action on the muscles, for both spastic and paretic conditions. Analagous mental and emotional states are also amenable to treatment on the Liver Meridian. This general dictum applies, of course, to all meridians — for the Ancients did not make the relatively sharp distinction between mind and body that is erroneously made by Western thinking. Although we can split, in words, the human make-up into body and mind, the two are empirically quite inseparable while there is life — they should not, therefore, be split in our thinking. True enough, one does tend to make various divisions as a matter of expediency — all the same it is important that we never lose sight of the fact that what we can verbally split cannot be empirically split. I shall be saying more on the subject of psychological disorders and their treatment later on in the text.

Seasonal Rhythms

In the previous lesson we discussed the 24-hour rhythm in the meridians; and the two-hour peak periods for each meridian. There is another factor to be taken into consideration when assessing the pulses. The organ energies have their yearly or Seasonal Rhythms of activity. That is to say, at each season of the year there are certain energy activities functioning more actively than at other seasons.

While reading this section, hold in your mind's eye the picture of the basic Five Element Diagram. You will recall that for certain purposes the Earth element is considered as occupying a central position, and is not associated with one of the traditional four seasons, but has (for some purposes) been attached to the end of Summer. The Ancients considered the functioning of stomach and spleen to have a throughout-the-year application and not as having the same range in rhythmic changes as the other organs.

In considering seasonal increased or decreased organ activity, we take the seasons as four — the traditional Spring, Summer, Autumn, Winter.

The Energies are at their maxima, as follows:-

SPRING	WOOD:	Gall and Liver
SUMMER:	FIRE:	Heart, Small Intestine, Circulation and Three-heater
AUTUMN:	METAL:	Lung and Large Intestine
WINTER:	WATER:	Bladder and Kidneys.

The first half of the year is characterized by Yang dominance of activity, which begins to stir at or about the Winter solstice and gradually increases in power until it reaches its height at Midsummer; then, after the Summer solstice Yin activity enters and steadily increases in dominance throughout the latter half of the year until mid-winter is reached once more.

The pulses on the left wrist, the Yang side of the body, are those associated with the first half of the year. That is, of course, if one considers the year to begin after the shortest day, when light is beginning to increase. The pulses on the right wrist, the Yin side of the body, are associated with the last half of the year — during which darkness is on the increase.

When Yang is on the increase the pulses of the left wrist should be stronger than when Yin is on the increase. The pulses of the left hand should always be stronger than those of the right; but they will be more so in the Yang half of the year than during the Yin half. The relative strengths between left and right must not, however, show too great a difference: this may be illustrated thus: Yang is looked upon as the husband and Yin as the wife; according to tradition, ''The husband rules the house.'' The husband should therefore be strong and the wife submissive.

If the husband is weak, chaos and disintegration follow; if the wife is weak, tyranny results (i.e. husband is over-dominant, or domineering).

There should be a fine balance of the cohesive and dispersive activities. The cohesive or organizing and focusing activity must always predominate and rule over the dispersive, separating and distributing activity, but always in just such a balance as to preserve life.

When he examines a patient the practitioner should not only glance at the clock and consider from the time-of-day angle whether a particular pulse should be strong or weak; he should also bear the calendar in mind, and consider from the season angle which organ energies should dominate.

As you will have realized from what you learned about polar changes, in Lessons 6, 7 and 8, it is at the extremes of activity that changes can be most easily accentuated (i.e. speeded up or slowed down). An individual's constitutional strengths and weaknesses will bear some consistent relationship to the season of the year and time of day when he was born. It is for this reason that one of my first questions to a patient, when writing out the case history, is: "When were you born?" Date and time?

According to the answer one gets one is able to form a preliminary assessment as to possible locations of strengths and weaknesses. To illustrate this, let us have an example.

Birth date and time: December 27 at 6 p.m. (Northern Hemisphere). (These notes are extracts from an actual case.)

According to Season Rhythm:

Water organs are at their Zenith
Fire organs are at their Nadir.

According to Daily Rhythm:

Kidney energy is at its zenith potential
The Large Intestine energy is at its nadir.

We estimate, therefore, that this patient at birth would have basic imbalances (either excess or deficiency) or tendencies in the Fire and Water organs: that is according to season potential. According to the time of day, these tendencies would be in the Water organ Kidneys, and Metal organ Large Intestine. The imbalance strengths may be in the organs themselves, their general functions, or in the associated tissues, and/or senses.

This means to say that whenever this patient is ill his particular way of being ill will conform to the pattern of his constitutional imbalances. The Chinese dictum "Every patient is ill in his own way — therefore treat the patient and not the disease" is exactly parallelled by the dictum of the great Dr. Samuel Hahnemann, the formulator of the homoeopathic medicine philosophy in the West.

In the case now under review the patient's own way of being ill, no matter what the illness, will involve primarily one or more or all of the following features, or shall we say that these organs, functions or tissues will figure in the primary symptoms:-

FIRE ELEMENT organs, parts of the body, tissues and sense:

Heart, Small Intestine, Circulation
and Three-heater

Tongue, Mouth, Face and Speech organs
Vascular system.

WATER ELEMENT organs:	METAL ELEMENT organs:
Bladder and Kidneys	Large Intestine
Ear and Hearing Sense	Nose and Smell Sense
Bones and Skeletal Systems	Body Hair
Hair on the Head, and	Mucous Tissue and Skin.
Sex Function.	

If, in this case, symptoms or disturbances occur in the other Elements' organs or tissues they will be ranked as secondary, even though they may be serious.

If we examine some of the illnesses from which this patient has suffered, and the ways in which these illnesses affected him, it will be seen how his basic pattern applied:

1. Rheumatic Fever which principally affected the heart and bones of the lower limb, in particular the knee articulation.

2. Measles: the feature here was an unduly prolonged high temperature, and the complication was in the ears and hearing. Though not deaf in the generally accepted sense of the word, it is characteristic of this patient that his hearing acuity diminishes whenever his tone gets low, or whenever he is ill.

3. At an early age he lost all his teeth, and the bony structure of his face is easily affected by changes of weather (especially winter cold winds) producing 'bony face ache'.

4. The vascular system is chronically weak; he suffers from haemorrhoids, and varicose veins on the leg.

5. Sexual tardiness of development, and several years impotent.

6. Chronic constipation for many years.

7. Almost without body hair, but luxuriant growth of head hair.

It is interesting to note that as regards this patient's eyesight — the fact that he wears glasses to read is not due to vision affected by any condition of the retina, muscle adaptation, long or short sight, but is due to slight ossification in one of the lenses.

In this case, it is not so much the actual Water Element organs, themselves, that seem affected, but rather the tissues associated with the Water Element, bones.

As regards the Metal Element, the organ itself, colon, mucous function, eliminatory function and, to some extent, skin, are all significant. (He has had ring-worm, boils in the nose and on the face, and his skin is easily broken.)

Some acupuncture schools consider the sexual system and function to belong to the Fire element. Though the "fire" element does figure strongly in the sex function, the primary relationship is with the Water Element organ, the kidney, as the general secernant organ of the whole body, together with all its systems. In other words, the secernant organ of the general (not vascular only) circulation has the closest possible relationship with the sexual function which is an eliminatory function — an entire system being excreted.

The foregoing notes should encourage you to think about your patients, their symptoms and their own ways of being ill, in quite a new light.

13

In cases of paralysis the opposite side or limb to the one affected is to be treated. In other words, treat the good side. Thus, for paralysis of the soleus muscle of the left leg one treats the right leg. The most suitable would be the sixth point of the Liver Meridian (VIII.6) on the muscle. Remember the rule: Supplement for paralysis and torpid states, or all hypo-activity. Moxa at VIII.6 would be my own choice of method, but massage or needle could as appropriately be chosen.

Spasm of this same muscle, the left leg would be treated on the left muscle, namely, the affected side. Treatment is draining or dispersive action. Remember the treatment rule: drain for pain, spasm, hyperactivity. Here one would not use a moxa, for with the moxa only supplementing action is possible. You have the choice of needle or massage. This point would be at medium depth for the needle, that is to say, from 1/2 A.U.M. to eight-tenths of an A.U.M. The needle is left in for up to 20 minutes, if needed. In all cases where the draining needle is used, it is well to leave the needle in until it almost falls out on its own.

In the case of uterine prolapse it would appear to me to be quite logical to use VIII.8 in supply action, because I associate a prolapsed state of the inner organs with insufficient activity of the relevant musculature. This also brings forward another treatment rule: when the site of the affection is on the trunk, or not at an extremity of the meridian path, a point is chosen at the knee or elbow. In this case, where it is a meridian of the leg, a point at the knee is chosen. This is the Water point of the Liver Meridian. The Water Element is associated with the sexual organs and function, and would therefore seem to be an appropriate selection.

Re-treating anuria at VIII.8, it would at once occur to me that the anuria would be due to muscle condition, since the meridian chosen is one that has special affinity for muscles and their states. Thus, if the condition is one of muscle spasm, draining action is to be used; if, on the other hand, the muscle state is one of underactivity, supplementing action is to be used.

VIII.8 is the Water Point of the Liver Meridian; one might therefore expect that, according to the Five Element method, this is a case of the Water organs showing an excess and the Wood organ, Liver, showing a deficiency: in which case, the proper treatment and point of choice would be VIII.8 in supplementing action.

Spasm and pain in the inner thigh musculature treated at VIII.8 is an instance (not of a distant point at the knee being used) of a local point being used. The correct polarity treatment would, of course, be draining action.

The Stomach Meridian (XI)

The Stomach Meridian is the second longest organ meridian, and has the distinguishing feature that it is the *only organ meridian with acupuncture points totally forbidden to any acupuncture treatment.* The location of these forbidden points makes the reason for their prohibition obvious. The points might as well be detailed now, memorized, and never forgotten. XI.9, the ninth point on the Stomach meridian, is on the external carotid artery — any pique here would be dangerous in the extreme: only a master of acupuncture might risk the use of this point, piqued very superficially indeed (and never moxa), in certain cases of pharyngitis, etc. It would be wise, however, to consider the prohibition as total and never risk using it. The point is bilateral.

The other forbidden bilateral point in XI.17, which is in the centre of the nipple, is a useful point to remember for its reference value in placing points both above and below it.

There are certain features about this organ meridian which not only make it one of the most generally useful of all meridians to know, but also it is one of the most interesting to study, on account of the wide range and variety of conditions treatable on this meridian. It has also on its path one of the greatest of all points, namely, XI.36, the Earth point.

Taking the points in numerical order they seem to fall naturally into three main groups: those on the face and neck; those on the trunk; and those on the lower limb.

Read the descriptions of the anatomical positions in conjunction with your study of the charts. You will notice that, where it has been expedient to do so, I have included on these charts some of the points of adjacent meridians. This should assist you in locating the points and appreciating the relative paths of the meridians. Had I done this earlier in the text it might have been confusing rather than helpful.

The three meridians of the leg have their first points close to the eye, the Stomach Meridian having the first point vertically below the centre of the pupil at the border of the orbitar cavity. This point is forbidden to the needle, but may be moxad. If you should need to moxa this point it would be as well to use the attenuated form in lieu of the artemesia cone. Use the joss stick, two or three applications sufficing for one treatment.

The second point just below the first (but the other side of the slight bony ridge that can be felt there) is a frequently indicated point for local symptoms. If you use the needle, remember that this point and all the points as far as and including the nineteenth point are to be piqued superficially. This means to a maximum of three-tenths of an A.U.M. In any case, it would not be possible to go much deeper than this at the majority of the points because of the underlying bone. On the thorax, however, care must be taken not to go too deeply with the needle.

XI.3 is just below the cheek-bone, nearly one A.U.M. from the nostril. The hollow will be felt. Compare what you feel with the chart illustration.

XI.4 is on the horizontal of the corner of the mouth, 1/2 A.U.M. from the meeting of the upper and lower lips, on the facial artery. This is an important point to consider in cases of affections of the eye musculature; as well as for use as a local point in facial paralysis, pain, spasm, etc.

XI.5 is on the lower edge of the lower jaw, in the facial artery groove. The depression is easily palpated and the facial artery may be felt pulsating.

XI.6 lies in the angle of the lower jaw among the masseter insertions. The depression is easily felt, and it will usually be found painful under pressure. The indications are usually local, such as inflammation, pain or neuralgia in the area.

XI.7 is one-third of the distance between II.18 and II.19, under the zygomatic arch, in the centre of the depression which forms upon opening the jaws. This point is forbidden to moxa. This is a useful deafness point, with or without tinnitus.

The path of the Stomach meridian now goes up as far as the horizontal hairline where, close to the frontoparietal suture, is the eighth point (see chart). Most of the European schools of acupuncture, based upon Soulie de Morant, refer to this as the First Point and trace the path of the previous seven points somewhat differently. I have a Chinese chart showing this as the first point, but it seems more logical to me to follow the Chinese tradition which places the first point at the eye. This eight point is forbidden to moxa.

The path now descends straight to the throat to the ninth point on the external carotid artery, anterior to the sterno-cleido-mastoidus muscle. See chart.

Two A.U.M. below the ninth point, on the border of the sterno-cleido-mastoidus, is the tenth point, XI.10. Remember this point for use in cases of whooping cough.

XI.11 is 1 1/2 A.U.M. lateral to the median line, just above the clavicle. This is a "knock-out" point in Judo and Aiki-do combat. If you use needles so remember that this point must not be piqued more than superficially. This point and the previous one (XI.10) are indicated in affections of the upper respiratory tract.

XI.12 is at the same horizontal level as .11 (above the clavicle) but 2 1/2 A.U.M. lateral to XI.11.

This now finishes the group of points on face and neck, and as we cross over the clavicle we begin the group of points on the trunk.

All the points on the thorax and abdomen are quite simple to locate, and the numbering of these points need represent no difficulty, provided you first

STOMACH MERIDIAN, XI

POINTS ON THE RIGHT LOWER LIMB
.31 to .41

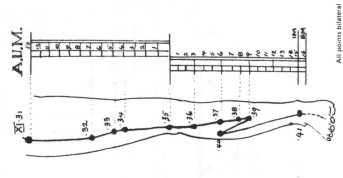

All points bilateral

STOMACH MERIDIAN, XI

POINTS ON THE HEAD
.1 to .10

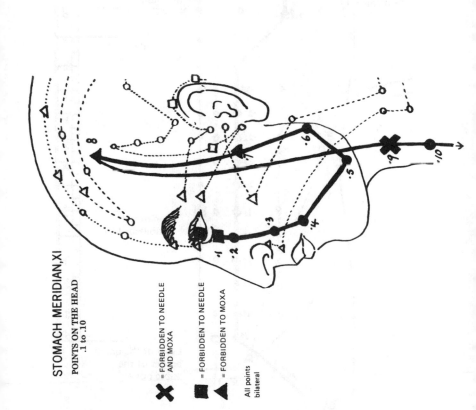

✕ = FORBIDDEN TO NEEDLE
     AND MOXA

▪ = FORBIDDEN TO NEEDLE

▲ = FORBIDDEN TO MOXA

All points
bilateral

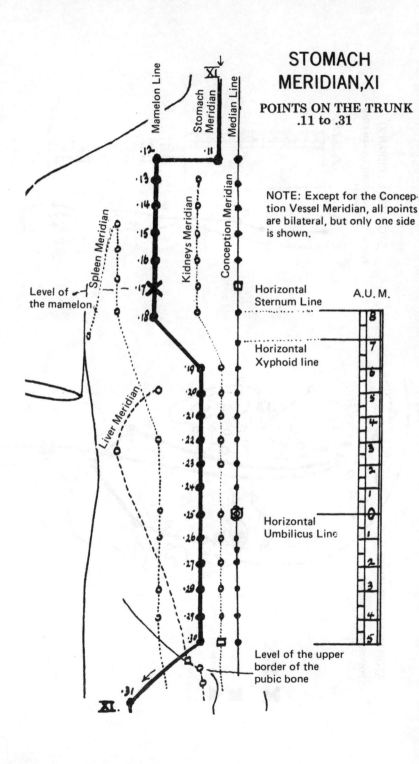

STOMACH MERIDIAN, XI

POINTS ON THE TRUNK
.11 to .31

NOTE: Except for the Conception Vessel Meridian, all points are bilateral, but only one side is shown.

A.U.M.

Mamelon Line

Stomach Meridian

Median Line

Kidneys Meridian

Conception Meridian

Spleen Meridian

Liver Meridian

Level of the mamelon

Horizontal Sternum Line

Horizontal Xyphoid line

Horizontal Umbilicus Line

Level of the upper border of the pubic bone

memorize one or two reference points.

XI.13 is just below the clavicle in the sub-clavian hollow, 1 1/2 A.U.M. vertically below .12.

XI.17 (totally prohibited to acupuncture action) is in the centre of the nipple. In the average male, this is in the fourth intercostal space. Draw a line from the thirteenth to the seventeenth point. The points between .13 and .17 are on this line in intercostal spaces. Thus, .14 comes in the first I.C.S.; .15 in the second I.C.S.; .16 in the third I.C.S.

This line, which you have just drawn, known as the 'mamelon line', is prolonged to the fifth I.C.S. Here is the eighteenth point, XI.18.

The path of the Stomach Meridian now descends at an angle towards the median line and crosses over the costal cartileges at the horizontal level of the sub-xyphoid fossa. This is at the same horizontal level as the twenty-first point of the Kidney Meridian (IV.21).

Our next reference point is at the horizontal level of the umbilicus.

XI.19 is where the path crosses the costal cartileges, and XI.25 is vertically below this at the level of the umbilicus. The points between these two are equidistant.

XI.19 at level of IV.21	XI.22 at level of IV.18
XI.20 at level of IV.20	XI.23 at level of IV.17
XI.21 at level of IV.19	XI.24 1/2-way between XI.23 and XI.25
XI.25 at level of IV.16	

In all cases of acute gastritis remember XI.21; indeed, this point should be considered as indicated in all indigestions and stomach disorders. Likewise XI.25 is to be treated in all cases of chronic stomach and intestinal troubles, especially in cases of chronic diarrhoea.

All the abdominal Stomach Meridian points would have local importance in the treatment of rectus abdominis spasm.

You will by now have noticed that local treatment for muscle spasm, paresis, or atony, is rarely at an acupuncture point in the belly of a muscle, but always close to the origin of the muscle concerned or at the tendon of insertion of the muscle. From the point of view of the Far-East 'polar' orientation this appears quite logical — for, to them, the two ends of the muscles represent the operative poles which, when there is stimulation, strive towards each other, causing contraction. To them it is obvious that the contraction will cease if the activated pole be discharged.

Below the umbilicus similar divisions occur as with the Kidney Meridian. For the next five points see chart. XI.30 is at the horizontal level of the upper edge of the pubis symphysis.

The Stomach Meridian path now leaves the abdomen and goes on to the anterior of the thigh; the thirty-first point (XI.31) is in the hollow formed near the apex of the angle formed by the sartorius and tensor fascia lata. This is at the same horizontal level as the great trochanter which, you will recall, is the reference point 13 A.U.M., above the level of the popliteal fold.

The Stomach Meridian path follows the interstice between the vastus externus and the rectus femoris as far as the patella. The upper border of the patella (which is 2 A.U.M. above the level of the popliteal fold) may be found to serve as a more convenient reference point for locating the Stomach meridian points, .32 to .34.

XI.32 is 5 A.U.M. proximal to (above) the patella
XI.33 is 3 A.U.M. proximal to (above) the patella
XI.34 is 2 A.U.M. proximal to (above) the patella
XI.35 is just below the patella, close to the lower border, on the lateral edge of the patella tendon.

3 A.U.M. below this last point we come to one of the most important of all acupuncture points: and I share the view held by many acupuncteurs that this point, XI.36, is to be ranked as one of the Very Great Points of Acupuncture. It is located in the depression between the tibia and the tibialis anticus muscle. For pique with the needle this is a moderately deep point, and it is admirably suited to moxa. This restriction must be remembered, however: on no account apply moxa to this point in the case of a child under the age of seven. Dr. Wu Wei Ping stresses this restriction.

The importance of this point may be more fully appreciated when one realizes that this point is the Earth point of the Stomach Meridian, and therefore also the Horary point; and remembering that the Earth organs' energy (stomach and spleen) has especial significance throughout the year. It is not so subject to seasonal rhythm, in quite the same way, as are the other Element organs.

A formula to be memorized as perhaps the most generally useful of all acupuncture formulae, is the combination of X.4 and XI.36, both in toning polarity. This formula is more than just an important gastro-intestinal tonic — it is used in all cases of hypo-activity anywhere in the digestive tract from one orifice to the other. This formula is often used in conjunction with other points to augment their effectiveness. Used as a single point, XI.36 may be used daily as a general tonic to maintain robust health; and, quite an important consideration, it may safely be used as a 'placebo' which will benefit the patient.

XI.36 uses as a distant point when there are symptoms on the path of the Stomach Meridian in the region of head, face, and neck (for example, in migraines).

XI.36 is also an ingredient in other formulae which will be given in subsequent lessons.

From XI.36 to XI.39 the meridian path goes vertically down between the tibia and the tibialis anticus.

XI.37 is 3 A.U.M. from XI.36
XI.38 is 2 A.U.M. from XI.37
XI.39 is 1 A.U.M. from XI.38

The Stomach Meridian path now turns back on itself at a hairpin angle and crosses to just the other side of the tibialis anticus muscle where, at the same horizontal level as XI.37, the fortieth point is located.

In order that the student may get some idea of the immense difficulty facing an acupuncture researcher in his efforts to decide which location to take as authoritative, I shall digress for a moment to give you but one instance. This concerns the location of the fortieth point, XI.40, which is an extremely important point, being the passage point from the Spleen Meridian to the Stomach Meridian.

In the 1959 text of his translation into French from the Chinese of Dr. Wu Wei-Ping, Dr. Lavier describes the fortieth point of the Stomach Meridian as 'on the antero-external aspect of the leg, posterior to the tibialis anticus at the level of point thirth-eight.'

On the chart, illustrating Lavier's translation, this point is shown as at the level of point thirty-seven.

In his book, "Memento d'Acupuncture Chinoise", Dr. Lavier gives a carefully detailed anatomical diagram showing the fortieth point as at the level of

STOMACH MERIDIAN,XI

POINTS ON THE FOOT
.41 to .45

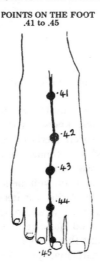

NOTE: All points are bilateral, but only one side is shown

point thirty-nine.

One writer — three different positions for the same point!

For the placing of this point I have taken as my guiding authority the official Chinese Charts printed and published in Peking for present-day medical students.

You will appreciate that I have gone to a great deal of trouble over many years to check and to countercheck the placing of acupuncture points. The locations given in this text are those which seem to me to be anatomically and most logical and most generally agreed upon by competent authorities.

XI.40 is coupled with VII.34 for constipation; and this coupling is to be added to the Nervous Disturbance formula X.4 and VIII.3, if the disturbance is severe.

The remaining points on this meridian can best be seen from the charts.

14

The Spleen Meridian (XII)

With this lesson we have now come to the detailed examination of the twelfth and last of the Organ Meridians, known as the Spleen Meridian (XII). This meridian, paired with the Stomach meridian, belongs to the Earth Element, which is particularly associated with connective tissue, the Reticulo-endothelial System, mouth, tongue and taste sense.

Spleen Energy has also association with mental development and intellectual growth. I make special mention of this last item because, in my own clinical experience, I have observed that certain psychological states, tardy developments and intellectual blockages respond quite remarkably to action on the Spleen Meridian points. One also notices that the Spleen Energy has peculiar affinity for certain aspects of sexual maturing, and "creative" processes on both physiological and the higher psychological levels. Spleen meridian points figure prominently in the treatment of genitalia malfunctions, both male and female. This has come to my notice over and over again.

The first point, XII.1, is at the medial ungueal angle of the big toe. This point is forbidden to Moxa, and, as regards the needle, this point must not be piqued during pregnancy. This prohibition to the needle in pregnancy also applies to the second point, XII.2, which is just distal to the metatarso-phalangeal articulation of the big toe, medial border at the meeting of the dorsal and plantar skins. The line of union of these two kinds of skin (dorsal and plantar) is easily traceable, and marks the exact path of this meridian to the fourth point. This second point is of special significance in the treatment of mental backwardness. It is the Fire point of the Spleen Meridian; the first point is the Wood point.

XII.3 is just proximal to the metatarso-phalangeal articulation of the big toe, inner (medial) border. This point has several features making it a highly important point.

XII.3 is the Earth point of the Spleen Meridian, and therefore also the Horary point; it is also the Organ or Source point. Among 'civilized' peoples this point seems to suffer more damage than almost any other point. If the reality of the meridian paths and the Vital Energies flowing through them were only more generally known and accepted, I feel convinced that the wearing of ill-fitting and/or highly unsuitable shoes would rapidly go out of fashion — and the abuse and maltreatment of the feet would be looked upon as a serious general health hazard.

XII.4 is one A.U.M. proximal to XII.3. This fourth point is the passage point linking the Stomach meridian to the Spleen Meridian. It seems strange to me that Dr. Wu Wei-Ping does not mention this point in connection with injury to the testicles: for it has been well known to the Japanese for many, many years as a remarkably effective point to relieve the pain caused by injury to the testicles.

As most people are right-handed, I shall describe the percussion massage as for a right-handed operator. The patient will be lying down or sitting. Take hold of the patient's right foot in your left hand so that your thumb is on the sole of his foot near the base of the big toe: grip firmly, and, if possible, hold the foot still by supporting it against your own left knee or thigh. Clench your right fist with the right forefinger first phalange extended. (You will strike with the distal end of this first phalange.) Touch the spot you are going to strike: draw the fist back about two inches, *not more than three inches.* Now, give three sharp blows, allowing two or three seconds between each. The blow is given by movement of the elbow joint — it is not intended to be a full-blooded punch from the shoulder!

SPLEEN MERIDIAN,XII

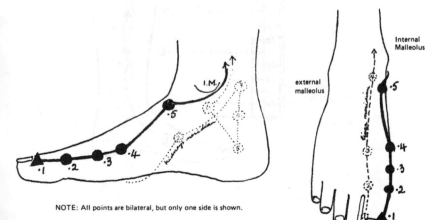

NOTE: All points are bilateral, but only one side is shown.

SPLEEN MERIDIAN,XII

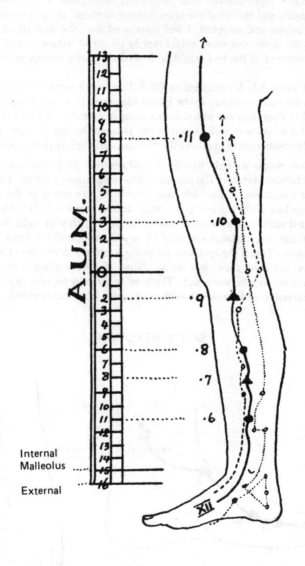

Internal
Malleolus

External

▲ = FORBIDDEN TO MOXA

There are occasions when a percussion, as just described, would be too heroic a measure: in such cases, one uses pressure as the alternative. I used this alternative when a boy had slipped off his bicycle pedal, and landed on the cross-bar, giving himself a nasty blow in the testicles. In his case, I pressed my knuckle firmly into the site of XII.4 and held it there while I counted seven; and then released the pressure steadily (though fairly rapidly). The effect was immediate. In a later lesson I shall be giving several more of these Japanese points for emergency treatments — they coincide with the Chinese points; it is the percussion technique that is peculiarly Japanese.

XII.5 is just anterior to and below the internal malleolus between the tendons of the tibialis anticus and extensor hallucis longus; in the hollow felt at the upper border of the lower band of the lower extensor retinaculum (see chart). This is the Metal point of the Spleen Meridian. This is a useful point in cases of atony of smooth musculature and of the elastic fibres of conjunctive tissue. Moxa at this point is indicated to impart tone and reduce articulation hypermobility. It is also used when there is ptosis of the abdominal and pelvic organs.

XII.6, one of the Great Points of Chinese Acupuncture, is four A.Ů.M. vertically above the most prominent part of the internal malleolus.

Dr. de la Fuye stresses the importance of this point for all female genital disorders and regulation of the menses: it should be noted, however, that this point is indicated in genital apparatus disturbances for both male and female.

Three important formulae incorporating this point should be memorized.

XII.6 + V.6 restores vitality in cases of weakness
and exhaustion.

XII.6 + XI.36 for all gastro-intestinal troubles.

XII.6 + X.11 for all uterine or ovarian disorders, and,
more generally, for all internal inflammations
and ulcerations.

Bleeding is controlled by the use of XII.6 as a single point; not only in cases of over-abundant menses and any uterine haemorrhage, but also in cases of bleeding haemorrhoids.

XII.7 is seven A.U.M. above the internal malleolus. Note
that this point is forbidden to moxa.

XII.8 is nine A.U.M. above the internal malleolus.

XII.9 is two A.U.M. below the level of the popliteal fold.
It can easily be palpated below the head of the tibia
between the insertions of the gracilis and semi-
membranous tendons. This is the Water point and is
forbidden to moxa.

XII.10 is three A.U.M. proximal to the popliteal fold, in
the interstice between the rectus femoris and sartorius.
The meridian follows the line of the sartorius to five
A.U.M. above .10, where the eleventh point, XII.11, is
located on the femoral artery. (Use the needle with
caution.)

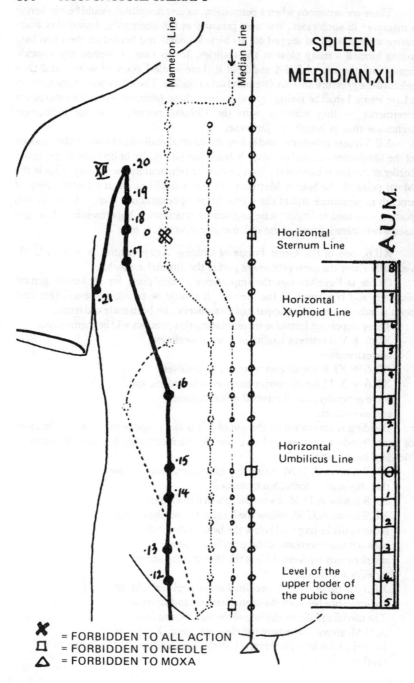

SPLEEN MERIDIAN,XII

A.U.M.

Mamelon Line

Median Line

Horizontal Sternum Line

Horizontal Xyphoid Line

Horizontal Umbilicus Line

Level of the upper boder of the pubic bone

✗ = FORBIDDEN TO ALL ACTION
☐ = FORBIDDEN TO NEEDLE
△ = FORBIDDEN TO MOXA

XII.12 is in the inguinal fold, vertically below the mamelon, and at the same horizontal level as IV.12. The Spleen Meridian points, .12 to .16 are all on this mamelon line:

XII.14 is one A.U.M. below the navel, at the same
level as IV.15 and XI.26
XII.15 is at the level of the navel, at the same
level as IV.16 and XI.25.
XII.16 is three A.U.M. above the navel, at the
same level as IV.18 and XI.22.

The Spleen Meridian path now continues upwards and laterally to reach the fifth intercostal space half-way between the anterior paraxillary line and the mamelon line; this locates XII.17.

The next three points are vertically above XII.17 in the 4th, 3rd and 2nd intercostal spaces, thus:-

XII.18 in the fourth I.C.S
XII.19 in the third I.C.S
XII.20 in the second I.C.S

The meridian path now turns back and down to the sixth intercostal space on the axillary line, where the 21st and last point is located.

Minor and Major Injuries

Now that you know the paths of the Organ Meridians, particularly those of the leg, it will no longer astonish you that so many people suffer all manner of aches, pains, and disturbances of the inner organs and their functions: rather, on the other hand, it may well be that you are amazed that more people do not suffer — especially when you observe such widespread follies, ignorances, and omissions exemplified in high heels, pointed toes, footwear cramping, torturing and distorting the feet; the astonishing little care that people seem to give to their feet; restrictive and/or unsuitable clothing for almost all parts of the body; tight hats, a whole host of minor injuries disregarded and left without any thought of treating them as worthy of treatment and quite serious injuries left incompletely treated.

A word or two about minor and major injuries. However slight the injury, cuts, bruises, tears, bumps or burns, some scar tissue forms. Each little injury may form such a relatively minute scar that, by itself, it can be looked upon as having insignificant effect on the total organism. But when there are several thousand of these trivialities the aggregate is no longer to be disregarded.

According to ancient tradition, scar tissue obstructs or diverts the flow of vital energy. A great many little obstructions and diversions have a cumulative effect upon the flow and equilibrium of vital energies, with repercussions on the internal organs and their functions.

After a fracture, little seems to be done for a patient when the plaster cast is taken off. I have known instances of patients even being advised not to allow massage to be applied. The result, then, is a more or less serious obstruction to the vital energy flow somewhere, and sooner or later there will be organic repercussions.

If a masso-therapist devoted his time to tracing systematically the Meridian paths on each patient, and applying massage of one kind or another throughout the whole length of each meridian, breaking down, dispersing and making flexible all scars and adhesions (muscular, fascial, tendinous, cartilagenous), he would be doing a very great service indeed towards the health of his patients.

By tradition the highest healing art is the preventive. That means to say, recognizing in the very early stages the potential sources of disease or sickness, and dealing with these in such a way that the disturbances never materialize as gross outward symptoms or symptom complexes.

It is only the inferior doctor who has to spend his time treating his patients for ills that he had neither the knowledge nor skill to prevent.

If they will not come to you until they feel ill, they have already robbed themselves of their best health opportunity; and, at the same time, they are being unfair to you, their practitioner, by making your task longer and more difficult than it need be; perhaps even imposing a task on you that you need never have had.

We look forward to the day when people while in good health will pay regular visits to their practitioner, in order to maintain their good health. I would suggest two visits, per annum, as the absolute minimum; preferably a visit at each season, i.e. four visits per year. In this way, a practitioner can keep an eye upon his patient over the years, getting to know and understand his patient at a really deep level.

We, in acupuncture, recognize that surgeons and others have their place — indeed, there are emergencies where surgery (or other heroic measure) alone will save a human life, limb or sanity. But after the ''make-do-and-mend'' or ''patch up'' performance has been completed, the patient should consult his own ''highest art'' practitioner, who may, in name, social and legal status, be only a humble masseur practising acupuncture-oriented physiotherapy, but whose long-term cultural value to mankind far exceeds that of practitioners working solely in the field of 'knife or syringe'.

Part four

THE VESSEL MERIDIAN

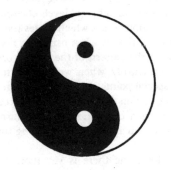

15

The Vessels and their Meridians

Up to this part of the book we have been concerned principally with the peripheral energy paths known as the Organ Meridians. The energy flowing through each of these superficial pathways is associated with its Source Organ.

One must realize that Vital Energy permeates every cell and tissue of the entire system: we should not therefore visualize it as flowing only through relatively confined pathways or series of pathways. We should try to visualize the main paths or meridians as the broad highways or main channels; in much the same way as the arteries and veins represent the main blood channels; and the large nerves represent only the main conduits of nerve energy. The whole system is supplied with blood (which is always on the move) and nerve ramifications forming a complex network covering the whole body. It is expedient to look upon the Vital Energy as having several different levels of circulation.

The deep inner circulation is that which unites the inner organs themselves. This is the circulation we deal with when using the Five Element Method. The surface circulation follows the pattern of the twelve organ meridians. It is this energy we manipulate principally when we deal with superficial, local, acute symptoms. At certain special points on this surface circulation (the only one we can reach directly) we take action to affect the deeper circulation.

Between the inner organ circulation and the surface circulation there are connective channels. The principal points for acting upon these are the Source Points.

In addition to the foregoing there is yet another system of conduits and reservoirs known as the Vessels. These have a special function. We shall now briefly discuss these Vessels and their meridians.

You well realize that as regards ordinary food intake and its combustion (conversion of food into energy) the rate at which one uses up energy is never constant; food is taken in at relatively long intervals -— perhaps every three or four hours during daylight. Thus, in order that there shall always be enough fuel available for combustion as and when required, there is the storage system in the body — the liver being a good example of a storage organ. Similarly, there are reserve systems for blood supply — so that emergencies of various kinds may be met.

According to ancient tradition there are Vital Energy reserve and regulatory complexes. That is to say, there are various reservoirs whose three-fold function is to accumulate, store, and regulate expenditure of energy excesses. First, the excesses have to be built up and preserved until required. Second, the proper level of energy flowing through the meridians and the whole system has to be maintained — this is the 'safeguard function' against accidental loss through injury or sudden increased expenditure. Third, changed or expended energy has to be collected prior to its elimination by appropriate gradual stages.

The circulation system involving these functions comprises what are known as the 'Eight Vessels'. In this text we shall be concerned in detail only with two of these vessels and their meridians (superficial paths). I have, nevertheless, given the names of all eight, together with a few basic items of information concerning them.

They are classified in pairs; and each of them is linked with a special superficial bilateral point on one of the organ meridians, at which the vessel energy may be controlled as a whole. These points are known as the Vessel Command Points.

Except for the two median vessel meridians, which are detailed in this text, the vessels have no superficial points exclusively their own—the Vessel meridian or superficial points are all points belonging to one or more of the Organ Meridians.

The two exceptions are the vessels known as the *Conception* and the *Governor* vessels. The meridians or peripheral path of the Conception starts at the centre of the perineum and follows the anterior median line up to the mouth. The meridian of the Governor Vessel follows the posterior median line from the tip of the coccyx, up the back, over the head, to the mouth.

The names of the vessels, their Command Points, and classification into pairs are in accord with Dr. de la Fuye's Treatise based upon Soulie de Morant.

FIRST PAIR

Vessel 1   The Vital Energy Regulator or De-obstructor
                    bilateral command point at XII.4

Vessel 2   The Yin Energy Conserver
                    bilateral command point at V.6

SECOND PAIR

Vessel 3   The Cincture or Girdle
                    bilateral command point at VII.41

Vessel 4   The Yang Energy Conserver
                    bilateral command point at VI.5

THIRD PAIR

Vessel 5   The Governor
                    bilateral command point at II.3

Vessel 6   The Yang Energy Accelerator
                    bilateral command point at III.62

FOURTH PAIR
Vessel 7   The Conception
                   bilateral command point at IX.7
Vessel 8   The Yin Energy Accelerator
                   bilateral command point at IV.6

The Conception Vessel Meridian

The command point of energy conception (or energy generation) is on the lung meridian at the seventh point, IX.7. This point is also the passage point on the lung meridian where the energy flows in from the Tenth Meridian. The linkage with "energy conception" and "oxygen" appears a logical one.

The peripheral path of the Conception Vessel meridian begins with the first point in the centre of the perineum. This point is forbidden to moxa. It is the only point on this meridian forbidden to moxa — though the eighth point has to be treated by moxa in a special way. Details of this special moxa technique are given in a later paragraph.

There are no points totally prohibited, and two points are forbidden to the needle, which we shall come to in due course. Reference to the chart for all the Conception points will make their location quite easy with great accuracy.

The second point is on the upper border of the pubis symphisis. This is one of the reference points for locating those on the lower abdomen. Although we have, in previous lessons, placed the points on Kidneys, Stomach and Spleen meridians before tackling the Conception, now that we have arrived at the detailed study of the Conception it will be found to be more convenient to look upon the Conception reference points as the best for the location of all points, using the "squaring" method, on the abdomen.

Divide the distance between Conception 2 and the center of the Umbilicus into five equal sections (5 A.U.M.).
Conc .3 is one   A.U.M. above .2 level of IV.12 XI.29
Conc .4 is two   A.U.M. above .2 level of IV.13 XI.28
Conc .5 is three A.U.M. above .2 level of IV.14 XI.27
Conc .6 is 3 1/2 A.U.M. above .2
Conc .7 is four A.U.M. above .2 level of IV.15 XI.26
Conc .8 is five A.U.M. above .2 level of IV.16 XI.25

This eighth point is in the centre of the umbilicus and is absolutely forbidden to the needle.

For the umbilicus to the tip of the xyphoid process there are reckoned seven equal divisions; or to the tip of the sternum, eight equal divisions. Thus we locate the next eight points:
Conc .9 is one   A.U.M. above .8 level of IV.17 XI.24
Conc .10 is two   A.U.M. above .8 level of IV.17 XI.23
Conc .11 is three A.U.M. above .8 level of IV.18 XI.22
Conc .12 is four A.U.M. above .8 level of IV.19 XI.21

Conc .13 is five   A.U.M. above .8 level of IV.20 XI.20
Conc .14 is six   A.U.M. above .8 level of IV.21 XI.19
Conc .15 is seven A.U.M. above .8 (at tip of xyphoid)
Conc .16 is eight A.U.M. above .8 level of IV.22 XI.18

As regards the Conception Meridian points on the sternum, these are taken as being on the median line at the point where the extension of the intercostal spaces would intersect that median line. Thus: -

Conc .17 fourth I.C.S. level (approx) IV.23 XI.17 (*Forbidden to needle*)
Conc .18 fourth I.C.S. level (approx) IV.24 XI.16
Conc .19 fourth I.C.S. level (approx) IV.25 XI.15
Conc .20 fourth I.C.S. level (approx) IV.26 XI.14
Conc .21 at the upper border of the manubrium, in the supra-sternal hollow.

The remaining three points are also simple to locate: -

Conc .22   is on the pomun adami. Although not forbidden to the needle great care must be taken—the pique is to be only very superficial, only just in the skin. This point must on no account be treated by either moxa or needle on children under the age of seven.

Conc .23   at the level of the Os Hyoidus.

Conc .24   the last point, is in the depression between the chin and the lower lip.

Points on the Conception Vessel Meridian

The special value of the first point on the Conception Meridian is for the resuscitation of a drowned person. A needle inserted here to a depth of one A.U.M. (in Supply Action) brings about an immediate urination which may save a human life. This helps raise the body temperature and stimulates the entire Vital energy. In the absence of a needle (for one does not always have equipment available in emergencies) sharp, sudden, deep digital pressure is to be applied at this point. There are other uses for this point, but owing to its location it would be wise to leave it alone, especially in the early stages of one's acupuncture experience. Never moxa this point.

Conception Points .2, .3, .4 and .5 have local symptom value; especially .5 which is a special point for all genito-urinary troubles. But take the precaution of not using a moxa on .3 or .4 if the Bladder is full.

Conception .6, known also as the Sea of Energy, is a very valuable point indeed to remember and to use. In common with so many of the abdominal points, it is eminently suited to moxa treatment. At this point (.6) the body's energy reserves are both opened up and rebuilt. Remember this point in cases of mental (nervous) depression and debility; also for intestinal and genito-urinary malfunction.

Conception .8, in the centre of the umbilicus, is a valuable point when vital energy seems low and there is general exhaustion. This point is *absolutely forbidden to the needle* and as regards moxa there is the special moxa technique referred to earlier. The umbilicus must first be filled with salt (preferably sea salt, though common salt will do) and the moxa cone is placed on the top of the salt. This point may be moxa'd very heavily — several applications at one treatment session.

This umbilicus point has good diagnostic value. Look long and carefully at the patient's navel; palpate both it and the surrounding tissues for texture. If the navel is deep, well-shaped and the surrounding tissues are strong and firm (not hard) prognosis is always good; as these are the signs of strong powers of resistance, good vitality reserves, and long life. If the navel is small, flat, shallow, then the vitality reserves are poor: if a pulsation is felt upon relatively light pressure and the surrounding tissues are dough-like, prospects are poor.

An excellent moxa formula for stimulation of vitality is the combination of Conception .6, .8, .12 and XI.25.

Deep and energetic massage from Conception .5 towards the solar plexus as far as .7 has long been known to the Japanese as having profound stimulating effect on the heart, lungs, abdominal aorta, and, in general, to stimulate free flow of Vital Energy.

Conception .12, also known as the "Harmonizer", has special value in that at this point mistakes of treatment can often be rectified. As its name indicates the overall effect of action at this point is to exercise a harmonizing influence upon the whole system, in particular over heart and lungs.

Two formulae to be memorized are: Conception .12 and XI.36 in cases of vomiting and diarrhoea. Also useful in sea sickness. Conception .6 and XI.25 for all maladies of the lower abdomen and uro-genitary system.

When acting on the Conception Meridian point below the navel, for treatment of genital affections, the nineteenth point (.19) is added.

Conception .10, .11 and VIII.13 is another formula with special effect on the gall bladder.

All the Conception points should be taken into account, of course, for any purely local skin and muscle symptoms.

Conception .17 is forbidden to the needle. This point has great diagnostic value. Spontaneous pain at this point is a warning of lung disorder or malady of one sort of another. The condition of the general circulation is also indicated here. If the point is spontaneously painful, or painful under relatively light digital pressure, this indicates a venous hydrogenoid constitution and tendency to sluggish circulation.

In acupuncture this point (Conc .17) is looked upon as the indicator of water-poisoning; e.g. when a patient's tissues are dough-like, flabby, hypotonic, and with oedemas. Use moxa at this point for all hydrogenoid conditions.

If a pulsation is felt at this point, but no pulsation is felt on the abdomen, it is considered by some authorities as a warning of danger of haemoptisis when moxa should be used.

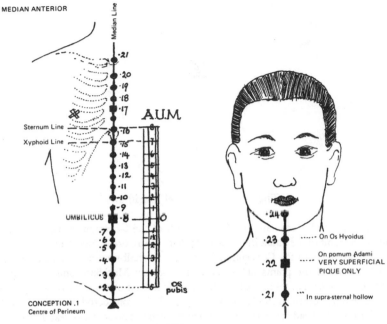

NOTE: MOXA AT .8 (Umbilicus Point) ONLY AFTER FILLING THE UMBILICUS WITH SALT.

Moxa at Conc .17 for all lung complaints, asthma, coughs, bronchitis, trachitis, angina, as well as fears and mental depressions.

Just as Conc .17 is the great indicator of water-poisoning, Conc .9 is the great point at which to treat water-poisoning.

Conception .15 has special action on the pituitary, and hence on the endocrine system as a whole, especially when used in conjunction with Governor .19. Note also that X.20 (last point of the Large Intestine) has special action upon the pituitary body. X.20 is sometimes known as "The Pituitary Point".

Conception .22 judiciously used can bring about quite spectacular results. This is the great point for the treatment of acute attacks of asthma; and for glottis and oesophagus spasm and all affections of the upper respiratory tract. When, for example, the "voice is lost" as a consequence of speaking for a long time, 30 seconds of stimulation massage at this point "brings the voice back" to full power and clarity. I have used it many times. Dispersion or sedative massage would naturally be used in cases of spasm or constriction.

Conception .12 with Conception .4 may be beneficially used for migraines and various psychological disturbances, mental alienations, etc.

16

The Governor Vessel Meridian

The Control (Command or Master) Point of the Governor energy is at II.3, the Wood point of the Small Intestine Meridian, a Fire organ meridian.

As we did with the Conception Meridian we shall now quickly run through the locations of the points of the Governor Vessel Meridian, and in the next section follow with notes on various therapeutic indications and uses of the points.

The only points on the Governor that could be considered difficult to locate are those on the head; even these skull points need not present any real difficulty if you have the A.U.M. notion well established in your thinking.

All the points on the Governor Meridian are on the posterior median line continued over the head to the top jaw.

The Governor Meridian begins with its first point at the tip of the coccyx.

.2 is at the sacro-coccygeal articulation.

.3 is in the depression between the spinous processes of the fourth and fifth lumbar vertebrae. With all the spine points the acupuncture point will be felt to be close always to the spinous process above the acupuncture point

.4	lies between the spinous processes	L3 and L2
.5		L 2 and L 1
.6	forbidden to moxa	D 12 and D 11
.7	*totally prohibited*	D 11 and D 10
.8		D 10 and D 9
.9		D 8 and D 7
.10	Forbidden to needle	D 7 and D 6
.11	Forbidden to needle	D 6 and D 5
.12		D 4 and D 3
.13		D 2 and D 1
.14		D 1 and C 7

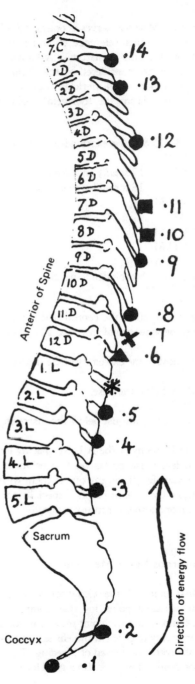

GOVERNOR VESSEL MERIDIAN

POSTERIOR MEDIAN LINE

SPECIAL POINT OF KUATSU: To stimulate heart action and stimulate kidneys, aorta, peritoneum, and brain. Use percussive massage.

▲ FORBIDDEN TO MOXA

■ FORBIDDEN TO NEEDLE

✗ FORBIDDEN TO ANY ACUPUNCTURE ACTION

Anterior of Spine

Direction of energy flow

This fourteenth point of the Governor Meridian serves as one of the reference points for placing the Skull Points — our other reference point being on the median line centrally between the eyebrows. This is anatomically known as 'the Glabella'. The Glabella point, however, is not considered by the Chinese as an acupuncture point belonging to the Governor vessel meridian, but is an extra-meridian (or "not-on-a-meridian") point. From the fourteenth point to the glabella is reckoned as 18 A.U.M.

From .14 to .15 measures 3 A.U.M. .15 & .16 are forbidden to moxa
From .15 to .16 measures 1/2 A.U.M.
From .16 to .17 measures 1 1/2 A.U.M. .17 *totally forbidden*
From .17 to .18 measures 1 1/2 A.U.M. .18 forbidden to moxa
From .18 to .19 measures 1 1/2 A.U.M.
From .19 to .20 measures 2 A.U.M.
From .20 to .21 measures 1 1/2 A.U.M.
From .21 to .22 measures 1 1/2 A.U.M.
From .22 to .23 measures 1 1/2 A.U.M.
From .23 to .24 measures 1/2 A.U.M. .24 forbidden to needle
From .24 to Glabella measures 3 A.U.M.

You will notice that if you take .19 to .20 as the central space, then either direction from this space we have the same sequence of spacings. This should help memorizing.

.25 is just above the point of the nose at the extremity of the nasal cartilege. This point is forbidden to moxa.

.26 is in the naso-labial groove just below the nose.

.27 is at the upper edge of the top lip, and

.28 is inside the mouth on the upper gum just below the insertion of the frenulum.

If you study the charts carefully and remember the A.U.M. spacing for these skull points, and actually locate and feel these points on two or three living subjects you will soon be able to place your finger on any one of them with great accuracy. It is rather important to know these skull points, especially the exact location of those forbidden to one action or another (or to any action).

Points on the Governor Vessel Meridian

In our very first lesson the first point of the Governor was listed for hemorrhoids. This is an extremely valuable point for that complaint. The treatment method of choice would be moxa, and the point may be moxa'd quite heavily. Our own clinical results seem amply to confirm the efficacy of this point whether the hemorrhoids are slight or severe, prolapsed or bleeding. The second point is also treated by moxa for hemorrhoids. Gov. .2 is also a good local point for dorso-lumbar neuralgia.

GOVERNOR VESSEL MERIDIAN

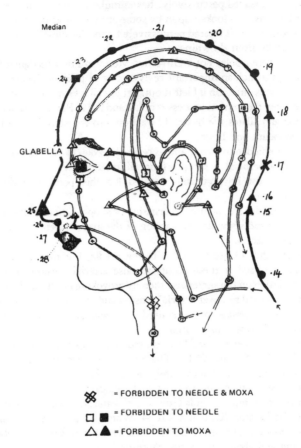

= FORBIDDEN TO NEEDLE & MOXA

= FORBIDDEN TO NEEDLE

= FORBIDDEN TO MOXA

Gov. .3, as with many points on this meridian, is suitable for the special percussion massage, as a resuscitation technique. Gov. .3 is used for genitalia disturbances, injuries or pains. It is used in combination with other points for a variety of conditions; local and distant — these can be found by referring to the repertory.

Gov. .4 has special action on the kidneys, genitalia and brain. Percussion massage may be used here beneficially as a general tonic. Needles, moxa and massage are all suitable. The point is used for insomnia, headaches and deafness (with tinnitus): and especially in conjunction with Gov. .20 for various prolapsed and ptosis states of the inner organs.

Gov. .5, massaged percussively, has stimulating action on the brain, aorta and genital organs. It is looked upon by some authorities as the most important of all revival points — it is treated percussively by the Japanese in cases of apparent death, especially from drowning.

I include here a point not a Governor Meridian Point recognized as such by the Chinese, but such an important revival point of Japanese Kuatsu that I feel it would be a serious omission if I left it out. Let us call it Gov. .5 bis. It is between .5 and .6; between the spinous processes of L 1 and D 12. Percussion here stimulates heart action and dilates the heart. The action also is a stimulant to the kidneys, aorta, peritoneum and brain.

Gov. .6 forbidden to moxa, and as regards needle (like all the spine points) the pique is only superficial — three or four millimetres only.

Gov. .7 must be accurately located for this point is forbidden to all acupuncture action.

Gov. .9 has this special use: Percussion or supply action at this point empties the gall bladder and stimulates the action of the liver, spleen, pancreas, stomach and the intestines.

Gov. .10 and .11 are forbidden to the needle, but moxa, massage or percussion may be used at these points to raise arterial tension. This is effected through the action on the surrenals, thereby provoking an afflux of adrenalin.

Gov. .12 is used to lower arterial tension and to dilate the lungs. Percussion, moxa, needle or massage may be used, and will be chosen according to circumstances and symptoms treated.

Gov. .14, between C 7 and D 1, is used as a component of the General Tonic Formula Gov. 14, X.4 and X.11. These three together augment the organism's powers of resistance; and may safely be used in conjunction with any other treatment to strengthen and re-inforce the efficacy.

As a general toning formula Gov. 14, X.4 and X.11 may be used on alternate days with the formula X.11 and VII.34. When using a general toning formula treatment this should be before noon — the best hours would be between five in the morning and about ten in the morning.

The alternation of these two formulae can be looked upon as giving a general stimulus and toning for the entire range of internal organs, especially liver, kidneys, intestines and stomach. Use moxas for preference.

Gov. .14 used percussively for resuscitation contracts the heart, aorta and pericardium and dilates the pulmonary artery. Thus, it serves as the revival point in cases of asphyxia.

Gov. .20 should be remembered as the Master Point for 'All that Falls' — it is indicated for all ptoses and prolapses. Gov. .20 is also indicated in extreme cases of nervous disorder and is used in conjunction with I.7 both in sedation action.

Gov. 25 at the extremity of the nasal cartilege is useful to sober up a drunk. But take note of the warning — stand behind the patient and hold his head pointing away from you, for the insertion of a needle here has the "sobering effect" of producing immediate vomit!

Part five

ACUPUNCTURE THERAPY

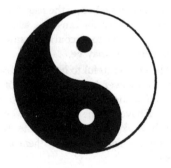

17

Draining Actions

You have already been given the general rule: "Drain for Pain," and, in the various repertories, lists of the points at which different pains are to be treated. This very general rule needs amplification — for quite a high proportion of patients come to a practitioner in order to obtain relief from pain.

In the first place it must be remembered that in principle all palliative treatment is to be avoided; but in cases where it appears expedient to palliate a patient's sufferings, this should be done only in full recognition that palliation is not cure; and, therefore, when one treats pain one is simply alleviating the pain in order to facilitate the basic treatment of removal of the causes of pain.

There are obviously emergencies when, if the pain is eased, the natural vitality will, of itself, deal adequately with the causes — and no more may be required than simple alleviation — so as to encourage nature to carry out her own healing work as unhindered as may be.

A patient may indeed be very grateful to have pain eased: and may look upon you, the practitioner, as a clever benefactor. Do not be deluded by flattery. Unless you are satisfied that the deep causes of the pain have been adequately attended to, you may well have left the patient in a worse condition than he was before — all you may have done is to remove the danger signal and left the cause untouched. In such a case the term "benefactor" would not be appropriately applicable.

You will also need to remember that acupuncture is not a cure-all — and that there are conditions for which acupuncture treatment is not suitable. For example, there are certain iatrogenic pains from which the only real relief is death itself; as, for instance, when nerve sheaths and other tissues have been irreversibly destroyed by some of the methods used for removal of cancerous tumours (e.g. radium, cobalt, etc.). Naturally, any acupuncteur will try to the best of his knowledge and skill to relieve pain; but he should know when a case does not belong in his field, and be willing frankly to admit this.

Consider very carefully, assisted as far as possible by pulse readings, exactly which meridians are affected and which points require draining action.

Never insert a needle into any spontaneously painful point, tumour, or swelling of any kind — and *never* into any other than an acupuncture point. Needles for the draining action are inserted at the nearest acupuncture points to the site of pain; and, if the painful area is a large one, several needles may be needed to encircle the area. Needles must be left in situ for at least half an hour or until the flesh no longer clings to the needle — in other words, until the flesh "lets go of the needles."

At each session it should be possible to close the circle in; proportionate to the reduction in size of the painful area — until eventually one or two needles only are needed. Not more than one treatment session per day should normally be given to a patient.

"Draining away" the pain is also draining away a certain amount of Vital energy. Remember the dictum, "Vital Energy must not be wasted." Some Supply Action must accompany the draining action. This can be done in more than one way.

If, for example, the pain is on the face close to the extremities of the meridians being drained, a Supply Action can be taken at the opposite extremity of the meridian. For this purpose, moxa would be the method of selection. The effect of this is twofold: (i) it would tend to draw the energy in that meridian away from the site of the pain towards the opposite end, and (ii) moxa brings in energy from outside in the form of heat. Alternatively, a toning formula can be used to help build up the body's reserves, and replace the energy resources.

The pulses may indicate a severe deficiency on one of the other meridians (not affected by the pain), so that the pain would be alleviated by drawing the excess out of the meridian in excess into the deficient meridian. In this case, encircling the painful area may not be needed at all, but only a re-balancing — taking Supply Action on the deficiency.

In every case, when treating for pain, Supply Action may appropriately be taken at X.4 or III.60 or at both. Use of one or both of these points ensures some balancing, toning action to whatever draining action is being taken elsewhere. X.4 is suited best to pain in the upper limbs and upper part of the body, and III.60 to the lower: in either case the whole system is affected.

Always close the series of treatments by a final session of re-balancing, according to the Five Elements, as indicated by the pulse readings.

Points for the Treatment of Pain

In the group lists which follow, I have collected under suitable headings the principal points applicable from which to make your selection. One would not necessarily use all the points quoted at one session; but, let's say, up to half a dozen at one treatment and a different lot the next, and so on. Always remember that it is the patient's vital energy you are manipulating, and you owe it to your patient not to weaken him by wasting his vital energy resources.

Make your selection with care from these lists: and you will easily be able to determine which points are to be drained and which supplied. For example, in Trigeminal Neuralgia, the local points for draining action would be selected from among III.7, VII.1, VII.11, VII.14 and XI.6, and the distant point for supply action is IX.7.

As another example: pain in the scapula, local points II.9, II.10, VI.15, and distant VII.25 and XII.7. In this example, however, supply action at XII.7 would not be moxa, for the point is forbidden to moxa.

Again, for headaches it is obvious that no practitioner in his right mind would put needles into all the points listed in any repertory. A careful selection would be made according to the location and type of headache, and taking all other relevant factors into consideration. For example, a frontal headache when treated between 3 and 5 in the afternoon might best be treated at the Bladder Meridian Horary Point, III.66, in Supply Action.

The Interaction of Mental, Emotional and Physical Disorders

According to Far-Oriental medicine philosophy it is axiomatic that one cannot split Mind from Body, and one cannot therefore treat the one without affecting the other. The patient is always to be considered as an organism-as-a-whole-in-environments. For again, it is axiomatic that environmental factors cannot be separated from a patient. In other words, a space with nothing in it is an absurdity; so too is a Thing with nothing surrounding it! The medicine philosopher teaches that treatment must always be given with a "wholeness" orientation.

In the West, in general, there is no medicine-philosophy in the Far-Eastern sense; and one finds "departmentalization" with, in consequence, attempts to treat the physical body, or even isolated parts of it, as if this treatment would have no effect upon the rest of the organism. Here and there one does come across medical men who think along lines in conformity with the facts of nature.

I have in mind three examples of such men: and I do most heartily recommend the earnest student to read (until he understands what he has read) at least one book by each of the following three authors:

(i)   Samuel Hahnemann, the book recommended is *Organon of Medicine* sixth edition translated into English by William Boericke, M.D., published by Boericke & Tafel, Philadelphia, 1952

(ii)   Georg Groddeck, M.D.,*Exploring the Unconscious* would probably be the most suitable single work to possess and study; and

(iii) Edmund Jacobson, M.D., *Progressive Relaxation,* University of Chicago Press, Chicago, Illinois.

The medicine philosophy of Samuel Hahnemann, as expounded in *Organon*, represents the nearest Western medicine philosophy to that of the Far-Orient that I have so far come across. Many passages in this book of his could as easily be imagined as quotations from some Far-Eastern text. In support of this there seems to be the fact of the widespread and profound appreciation of Hahnemann in such countries as India. The suitability of a "marriage" between Acupuncture and Homoeopathy was envisaged by Dr. de la Fuye, who made what was probably the first attempt to bring these two therapies together. Dr. de la Fuye, however, was not a philosopher; and his efforts at the 'match-making', creditable though they must undoubtedly be considered, cannot be looked as more than a beginning. There is a great deal of work to be done by anyone well versed in both Homoeopathic and Acupuncture principles.

It is clear that Groddeck thoroughly understood the inseparable relationships of body-mind: his contributions to the literature of psychoanalysis are world renowned. A careful study of Groddeck will bring a practitioner near a valid and sound knowledge of what physical symptoms to treat for certain related mental or emotional disorders, and vice versa, how to approach psychologically and treat analytically related physical conditions.

Although Dr. Jacobson did not (as far as I am aware) set out to demonstrate body-mind unity of function, he did, in fact, experimentally demonstrate (as an indisputable fact of observation) that *all thought processes and mental states co-exist with related muscular activity and tension:* and, in practice, if a therapist is able adequately to affect the muscle tensions and activities he will ipso facto affect to the same degree the thought processes and mental states.

As regards the treatment of psychological disturbances by acupuncture, and what mental conditions are likely to respond to acupuncture, de la Fuye makes it quite clear, in his Treatise, that mental cases arising out of cerebral lesions and tissue degeneration are, for the greater part, not treatable by acupuncture: but the mentally backward, misfits, maladjusted, neurotics (particularly cases of anxiety neuroses) and depression cases, respond well to the needles. He is careful to add that there are also cases which respond to acupuncture by "suggestion."

Dr. de la Fuye emphasizes (and I reiterate and emphasize this also) that a practitioner must be supple in his outlook, and not seek at all costs to make any one method triumph over all others. Above everything else the practitioner must have the desire to heal the patient. And, he says, it would be evidence of narrow-mindedness to reject a priori a synthesis of acupuncture and other methods on the grounds that such a synthesis of methods is not in strict accord with the ancient tradition of 'pure' acupuncture.

The ideal therapist is one whose spirit is pliable enough, and whose knowledge is broad enough, for him to use at one and the same time the quintessence of all known reputable methods. There is no need for conflict between adherents of different acupuncture schools, or different methods: on the contrary, the ideal is a combining of them all into the one and only valid therapy, namely, the one that heals.

As far as I have been able to understand Far-Eastern medicine-philosophy and practice the Far-Eastern practitioner never relied upon acupuncture as the sole means of effecting a cure. It was always accompanied by some other supporting treatment according to the patient's needs — be it by diet, exercise, baths, manipulation, herbal remedies, lotions, liniments, potions, packs, plasters and poultices.

I hope it is understood that when I talk about treatment of the psyche I am not thinking in terms of modern Western psychiatry (with its use of shock and drugs) but rather in terms of psychoanalysis and systems derived therefrom.

Anyone who has been through the two years of psychoanalysis considered in some quarters as the necessary qualification to practise analysis (that is to say, not less than 200 hours of analysis spread over two years) will be only too painfully aware that:

(a) Psychoanalysis, from the patient's point of view, can be a very expensive way of having the 'psyche' treated; especially as a beneficial outcome is by no means certain.

(b) Whether it is in the end successful or not, psychoanalysis seems inevitably to be accompanied by a great deal of emotional torment and distress.

It is desirable, therefore, that there should be some alternative and far speedier method of "resolving analytical problems." But this does not mean to say that I look upon Chinese Acupuncture *by itself* as an alternative to psycho-analysis in all cases; but rather do I intend to convey that a knowledge of an judicious use of the Chinese Acupuncture points can serve as an extremely useful technique for bringing about much more rapid results without torment, and with greater predictability.

If one wants to find classical justification for linking psychoanalysis with acupuncture, I could draw your attention to the passage in the Nei Ching dealing with the interpretation of dreams. Several thousand years before Freud, the Chinese recognized that dreams represent a mechanism for symbolic wish-fulfillment.

You should have no difficulty in appreciating that any disturbance in the flow and balance of the "Life-Force," with its two poles Yin and Yang, manifests itself as a disturbance more or less severe in both psyche and soma.

In my own analytical experience and physiotherapy and acupuncture practice, I have found such overwhelming confirmation of Groddeck's findings that I feel it is beyond dispute that an habitual state of mind sooner or later will show itself in analagous or related states of body.

As an example: fear, whether acute or chronic, can quite suitably be labelled a "state of mind"; there is also no disputing the fact that fear has physical manifestations. Fear will not always manifest in the same way; we can divide the manifestations of fear into two broad categories, Yin or Yang.

In the one type, Yin, the person goes *limp* with fear; rooted to the spot, out of a feeling of utter weakness and inability to act. There is an urge to flight, but no ability to do so. Muscles seem paralysed—there may be incontinence through vesical paresis—there may be diarrhoea, etc.

When treating a patient manifesting a psychological state of fear of this kind, we work on the basis that if any physical disturbances happened they would be in line with those just listed; and, even if these physical manifestations are absent, we select an acupuncture point or points at which one would treat such manifestations should they be actually present. "Yin" fear would be treated as for incontinence through vesical paresis, and/or diarrhoea, and/or extreme weakness. Fear of this "Yin" kind reflects a depletion of vital energy, deficiency of heart. One might treat as for paralysis of the muscles of the larynx (the person wants to cry out but is unable to make a sound).

The other type of fear, "Yang," instead of making the subject limp with fear, makes him stiff with fear. Instead of the urge to flight, there is the urge to fight, an aggressive urge accompanied by indecision. Physical symptoms, if they occurred, would also include incontinence: but this time incontinence due to vesical spasm. The urge to aggressive action tenses the muscles. So, for this category, a point or points would be chosen as if those physical manifestations were actually present (to some degree they certainly will be). That is to say, one would treat as for cramps, spasms, convulsions even, and select such points as III.62 (incontinence due to vesical spasm) II.3 the anti-convulsive point, or VIII.3, VII.34 and VII.40 for painful cramps.

Closely associated with fear is anger: which, from a psychoanalytical viewpoint, is often looked upon as an aggressive manifestation of fear. According to Groddeck and others, also confirmed by our own experience, suppressed anger leads to chronic tenseness in the arm and shoulder musculature; to neuritis pains in the arms, and so on. One of the points at which these physical symptoms would be treated is V.9

Popular expressing will give valuable clues — as, for example, one often hears a person say, when referring to some circumstance that makes him angry, "How galling." Such an exclamation from a patient would at once turn our minds to the Gall Bladder meridian where we might expect to find some disturbance of excess or congestion.

In the course of psychoanalytical sessions, or during a physiotherapy treatment, if one listens attentively and sympathetically to a patient's conversation it may become quite clear that this person's difficulties arise out of being too rigid in his ideas, being over-conventional, placing a reliance upon tradition, authority, etc.; and not having sufficient fluidity or flexibility of ideas.

Rigidities on the level of the psyche will tend to manifest correspondencies on the level of the soma. Fixed ideas are all too often the precursors of fixed or stiff joints or muscles. Even if muscular or articular rigidities are not yet actually present, we would select points to treat as if the physical rigidities were already there.

Rigid narrow minds, over-conventionality, and the kind of stubbornness and obstinacy that refuses to change or to re-evaluate prejudices, etc. would be treated as for arthritis, muscular rheumatism, fibrositis, and so on. One would, of course, consult the pulses for confirmation.

There is another point generally overlooked by practitioners (of any form of therapy) to which I must draw your attention. One must be prepared for the unexpected. Every therapist, in any field, will come across cases where to all appearances the patient's needs are so-and-so, and to such-and-such treatment he should respond. It has always worked before — is generally considered the correct treatment for the case — but, for some reason, exactly the opposite happens! The therapist may never know why. One does come across some quite astonishing and wholly unexpected reactions to acupuncture treatment — for which we might well be at a complete loss for an explanation. I will quote just one example to illustrate what I mean.

In strict accordance with the symptoms and the pulse indications, several points were treated in order (among other things) to calm down the action of the heart — but the patient responded as if the heart had been very much over-stimulated by the treatment. One of the points treated was on the Bladder Meridian, III.8. The response was so distrèssing that immediate action had to be taken to antidote this. It occurred to me at the time (and was later confirmed by psychoanalytical observation) that the puncture on the head had brought about this heart reaction, but, nevertheless, not because the choice of point was wrong, but simply because a needle was used on the head. In all probability, if any point on the head had been used the reaction would have been the same: Why? It was because the symbolism of what was done brought about the reaction, rather than the actual pique doing it. *For the symbolism brought about a reaction in the patient's psyche which was the polar opposite of the physical reaction which would ordinarily have occurred.* In other words: the stimulus of the symbol was stronger than the physical stimulus, and thus not only nullified the physical stimulus but overpowered it sufficiently to aggravate the opposite. If you study Groddeck you will soon realize how this sort of thing comes about.

Many worries, anxieties, power-complexes, and sexual problems are linked with constipations, haemorrhoids, ear, nose, and throat troubles.

In my closing remarks for this section, I give it as my carefully considered opinion that in acupuncture we have one of the most powerful of all therapy methods for the treatment of psychological disturbances so far discovered by man.

Classification of Pulse Readings

In one book in my possession, a learned Indian doctor lists no less than 66 different kinds of pulse beats, which, he says, are only the principal differences to learn to recognize in order to diagnose accurately. Sensitivity to the pulse so refined as to enable a practitioner to differentiate that number of pulse beats requires years of experience and guidance by a master of the art. In the Nei Ching you will find relatively few broad categories of pulses — expressed in terms difficult for a Westerner to visualize. Which of us, in the West, for example, would know when a pulse was like a leaf floating on the water? Or like scraping a piece of bamboo? Or like a string of pearls?

Some classification, however, we must have, in order that we may assess whether the pulse beat that we feel indicates fullness or emptiness, Yang or Yin. Likewise we need to have sufficient broad divisions of other signs of fullness and emptiness.

In general, the signs of fullness (or excess) are these: a pulse/respiration ratio greater than 4/1; the pulse being full, or hard, or rapid, strong or bounding: heat, redness: pain, whether sharp pain or dull ache: breathing energetic, forced, deep, or rapid: mental and emotional over-excitement: hyper-activity, restlessness: swelling: strictures, spasms, cramps, contractures: constipation; scanty perspiration: both pulse and respiration too rapid, though in the proper ratio of 4/1: general flesh texture too firm or rubbery or stringy.

The excess or hyper-activity can mean that the Vital Energy is being used up too rapidly, and it may be then that the activity needs calming down. Fullness or excess does not necessarily mean that there is a surplus to be drawn off.

The indications of emptiness or deficiency are these: a pulse/respiration ratio less than 4/1; the pulse being small, soft, slow, weak: cold, pallor: torpidity, numbness and tingling, insensitivity, paralysis: breathing slow, weak, shallow: mental and emotional depression: lassitude: pruritis: flaccidity, absence of 'tone' to the flesh: cold: general flesh texture limp, dough-like, puffy: excess sweating: diarrhoea: pulse and respiration both too slow, though in correct ratio the one to the other. These are the main indications requiring Supplementing, Supply or Toning action.

When assessing your patient, do so as far as possible in silence; but, of course, listen with patience and sympathy to the sufferer's own descriptions of what he feels: and do not despise your own intuition.

The better your own state of health, the more reliable will be your own intuitive assessment. It is of the utmost importance that you, yourself, be in a first-class condition of health — be a living example of what you practice — carry your measurement standards (norms) around with you in living form in your own body and mind.

The Main Acupuncture Rules

Acupuncture action, whether needles, moxa or massage, as by now you well appreciate, is to be taken only after careful assessment—and then only and always according to certain strict rules. Only one treatment formula is to be used at any one session. One does not jumble up the treatment rules and apply several at a session haphazardly. At each treatment session or visit you are naturally free to apply whichever rule you select as appropriate — but not two at a time.

It will be useful for both memorizing and reference if you now have the main rules summarized.

1. *The Five Element Rule:* As indicated by the pulse readings take supply action with massage, needle or moxa on the appropriate deficiency/deficiencies using for this purpose the Element Points, Passage Points, Source (Organ) Points or Horary Points. This is the highest method: use it whenever it is possible: always conclude a treatment series with it.

2. *A Single, Distant, Special, Master or Great Point:* Among the best examples of this is the use of such points as X.4, XI.36, XI.45, VII.34, VII.41, VIII.3, II.3 etc.

Distant points may be used:
(a) unilaterally
(b) bilaterally (if, for example, the symptoms are median or bilateral)
(c) the special application of the single point at a distance is in the use of the point at the opposite end of a meridian — the use of the ''nail'' points when the *affection is on the face*
(d) a distant point on both upper and lower limb coupled bilaterally.

3. *Action at the Acupuncture point or points closest to the symptom or affected part.* This is done by:-

(a) One or two local points being chosen on the affected meridian

(b) Several local points encircling the affected area

(c) Several points in a line on the affected meridian.

4. Combining (2) and (3) gives us the Local and Distant Rule. In general, when selecting an appropriate distant point to use, bear in mind that if the condition is acute a great point would be chosen on a limb, on the head, or anterior of the trunk; but if the affection is chronic the 'distant' point would be selected from among the vesical Element points.

5. If a whole limb or segment of the body is affected, points are selected: -

(a) Both anterior and posterior at the same approximate level. I have nicknamed this the "fore and Aft" rule. As an example, in genitalia affections, menstrual pain, etc. one would use the sacral foraminae points (III.31-34) posteriorly and anteriorly the Conception points .3, .4, .6.

(b) Coupling related (paired) meridians (i.e. the "Inside-Outside" rule), as for example using the formula X.4 coupled with IX.11.

6. *Special Formulae*

This can be looked upon as an extension of the use of the Single Great Point. In the course of several thousand years' experience the Ancients and their descendants discovered that certain groupings or combinations of points had very powerful specific effects. Into this category would come the various "tonics" and other formulae. You have been given important formulae in the various lessons.

Learn to work without using the charts (the best permanent chart is your own body and brain) and without elaborate equipment. An array of gadgets and instruments may have showmanship value — if you find such to be necessary — but remember all your books, charts, needles, gadgets, electronic or other devices may be lost, left behind, destroyed, taken away from you, and so, but while you are able to use your fingers and your brain you can practice acupuncture.

Treating a Patient

1. What is this patient's present energy pattern? Or, in other words, are there any pathological excesses and/or deficiencies—if so, where are they?

All your questionings, all your observations, what you see, smell, hear and feel, are all directed towards the discovery of this patient's energy pattern and to assess to what extent there are departures from normal requiring treatment.

Feel the pulses — note breathing and P/R ratio — is there heat or cold? Hyper- or hypo-activity? Excess colour or deficiency of colour in complexion, urine, stools, etc.? Is the flesh firm or limp? Is there tenseness or flaccidity? Where?

2. What is the most efficient way of bringing this pattern to normal?

For this you will need to know what kind of action has particular effect at any chosen point. Remember always that it is an energy pattern you are dealing with; and it is energy that you are manipulating. You are not concerned to name and to classify disease germs! Your action is not directed towards any single symptom, let us say for example such as 'decreasing alkilinity in the urine' per se — always your mind is focussed on the energy pattern and how to alter that. Having decided at what points action is to be taken, and in what polarity it is to be given, and what technique is most suitable, then and then only do you act.

The Glands of Destiny

The Endocrine Glands have so aptly been called 'The Glands of Destiny'. It was not until after I had read (and pondered on) a work on Tibetan medicine philosophy that I really began to get the general feel of the Far-Orient medicine-philosophical attitude towards the endocrine system; and to understand to some degree the relationships of these glands to one another. The Tibetan Chi-Schara-Badgan doctrine classifies these glands rather differently from the generally accepted Western classification.

My own opinion (largely intuitive but which, alas, I am not able to back up with quotations from authoritative texts) is that the Chi Schara Badgan medicine philosophy should be considered as a relatively pure representative of the basic medicine philosophy underlying all Far-Orient medicine.

Although this book is on Chinese Acupuncture, I do not feel it is out of place to list the "glands of destiny" in the Chi-Schara-Badgan order, which appears thoroughly logical — for it is in this order that they are developed in the embryonic branchial arches and oesophageal pouches.

I include in the list the post-branchial bodies (or ultimo-branchial bodies) even though they are not recognized in Western Medicine as of any significante — they disappear within the first few weeks of embryonic development. It fills me with wonder that the Ancients could, without microscopes, have known so much about these particular bodies, invisible to the naked eye; especially as the opportunities for examining a human embryo (from two or three days old up to two or three weeks old) would be very few and far between. Acupuncture is not concerned with the post-branchial bodies.

The Chinese Acupuncture Points which I give here for treating disturbances of the endocrine system are in the main based upon information collected by the late Dr. de la Fuye.

The "glands": pituitary, pineal, thyroid, tonsils, parathyroid, thymus, post-branchial bodies, surrenals, and testicles/ovaries. Points are not given for the pineal nor post-branchial bodies.

PITUITARY BODY

as a whole: Governor .16 .18 .20
anterior lobe: IV.11 IV.13 VII.37
posterior lobe: XII.5 III.60 Governor .11

THYROID

hyperthyroidism:

XI.9 Conception .15 .23
III.15
Governor .14 .20 I.7
VIII.2 X.4

hypo-thyroidism:

(depressions, physical fatigue,
asthenia, impotence, etc.)
Governor .14 .20 IX.9 .10 IV.7
Conception .6 VI.3 and X.4

TONSILS

hypo- hyper-activity, drain
or supply, according to symptoms:

VII.20 .21 III.10 .11 .12 .54
XI.9 .6 X.3 .4 .11 .17 IX.11
VI.1 .3 .17 II.14 .15 .16

PARATHYROIDS

hyperactivity:

III.11 .58 VII.30 XI.36

Hypo-activity:

II.3 V.6 VIII.2 .3 Conception .15

THYMUS

XII.2 III.11 VII.34

SURRENALS

hyperactivity:

XII.6 V.7 III.47

hypo-activity:

IV.7 III.47 XII.6 Governor .11
.16 .18

TESTICLES

hyperactivity or
hypersecretion:

XI.30 Conception .3 .4
III.60

hypo-activity or
insufficiency:

IV.11 Governor .3 .4 .5
III.47

OVARIES

hyperfolliculine:

IV.2 IV.13 VIII.3 XII.6 Conception .4

hypofolliculine:

IV.7 .13 III.67 VII.37 XII.6

Dietary Regulations

In one of his books Dr. Nyoiti Sakurazawa makes what, at first sight, appears to be a somewhat arrogant remark. He says that acupuncture never fails, and if after treatment the patient does not get well, or has a relapse, it is not the fault of acupuncture but the patient is wrong. A very similar remark was made by the great Samuel Hahnemann as regards homoeopathy. He says that if, after the correct dosage of the simillimum has been given, the patient does not get well or has a relapse then it is a sure sign that there is some external circumstance or habit that is keeping the diseased condition alive, and a cure is not to be expected until and unless that circumstance is altered. This is indeed very true in relation to acupuncture treatment. We assume, of course, that the points have, in fact, been correctly selected, located and treated.

Among the most important of all external circumstances and habits that militate against complete cure is diet. You may have already discovered that patients appear unwilling to alter individual diet habits one iota; but expect the practitioner to get their health up for them, without the patient's having to do a thing about altering diet (or any other) habits.

Do not expect your patient to be cured so long as faulty diet persists.

When I gave a patient a diet sheet I used to have the direction worded thus: "Follow this diet as thoroughly as you are able in your present circumstances." But I found that this very sentence was used as the excuse for not making any alteration at all. Now we have to tell the patient: "This is the regimen for you, and this must be strictly adhered to in every detail." No compromise!

After many years of research and experimentation with many different diets (personally carried out and observed) I come to the conclusion that the basic foods of diet are few and simple. The diet regimen which we, as a family, follow very strictly is based upon the Far-East medicine-philosophic principles. If you wish to enjoy optimum health you will follow these out yourself; and insist that your patients, if they want to get the optimum results from treatment, also observe these simple rules.

1. *Consume no more than is sufficient for health:*

Far too many people eat too much, too often. But this is not necessarily because of greed or self-indulgence. The body requires certain ingredients in proper quantity, quality and relative proportions. If one or more of these required ingredients has been removed from the food by refining the body remains in a permanent state of hunger for that very ingredient, and will therefore go on eating (long after the stomach and all other organs complain) in a desperate attempt to find that missing element. Thus, in order to get that which is missing, the body will take in an appalling excess of some other ingredient which, in proper proportion would be correct for health, in excess becomes a killing factor.

2. *Masticate:*

Food should be chewed until it almost disappears without needing to be swallowed. The food should just disappear down the gullet imperceptibly. The Med-Phil reason for this is that matter cannot be integrated (absorbed and made part of) into a new organism or system until it has been completely de-polarized. The de-polarization is effected by breaking up the elements into very small particles all of which must come into contact with the de-polarizing factor — saliva. Every particle of food that is swallowed without being de-polarized acts as a potential or active disturbing and/or disruptive factor.

3. *Three items that must be eliminated from the diet:*

Common salt

This is not easy when one considers that common salt is included in so much tinned, preserved and packeted foods. Common salt is a killer. Use sea salt instead. You may eat as much sea salt as you wish; it will never provoke excessive thirst nor cause the many distressing symptoms that follow on excessive common salt intake.

White sugar

Cane or beet sugar in the refined white state is to be cut right out of the diet. Again, this will mean steering clear of a wide range of tinned and preserved foods.

White flour and all refined cereals

Unrefined whole grain or whole flour, being the natural food for man, should form 80% (by weight) of his diet.

4. *Avoid:*

All chemical and synthetic 'foods' and drugs.

All foods containing artificial colouring and flavouring.

All foods that have been subjected to sprays, chemical fertilizers, etc.

All processed, battery-bred, caponized, etc. foods.

5. *Choose:*

For the 20% of your intake what is other than whole grain.

Fruits and vegetables in season, these being eaten raw or cooked.

Meats that are red, lean, compact (e.g. organ meats, lean beef, etc.) in preference to fatty meats (e.g. pork).

Free-run hens' eggs and poultry.

Cheeses.

Pulses, beans, peas.

Sea Foods: Fish, and edible sea-weeds (e.g. Caragean, Kelp).

Herbs for flavouring.

6. *Drastically cut down liquid intake:*

Urination per day should not exceed four times. This is the best guide as to the correctness of the amount of drink.

Your own daily health "barometer" is the stools. In good health these should be: long, soft, formed, floating, golden brown, and without unpleasant odor.

7. *Live simply:*

Work is not the sole aim and purpose of living; living should be a joy, together with all the activities of life. A joy shared is a joy doubled.

This lesson, the final one of this study has been the hardest to write, for there is still so much left unsaid. What you have been given is sufficient for you to start well on the road to becoming an efficient practitioner. You have had the basic principles and essential material to treat with confidence in a thoroughly sound manner; enough indeed to keep you going for several years. It is my earnest hope that you will not let your acupuncture studies progress no further than this book, but that as time goes on you will continue investigation, study and research on your own account.

If you will use, in the present, that which has been accumulated and handed on to you from the past culture, and, if you can, add something to it and pass it on for the benefit of future generations of mankind you will indeed be working and living in accordance with the highest ethic — and effort in this book will not have been in vain.

Pulse Correction

Having studied the foregoing, I will now give you the formulae for Pulse Correction of the patient's immediate condition. In other words, if you find that the Heart Meridian is FULL and the Liver is deficient then you will peek point 4 of the Liver, point 10 of the Lungs, then point 5 of the Heart.

Retest the pulses checking that a difference has been made. Always peek the Deficiency. NEVER drain the heart, remembering that the Lungs are the Mother of the heart. These two organs are life itself, and may not be disturbed—nly corrected.

The work of this book is to give the student a basis of knowledge, for there are Master points not so far mentioned; only practice of the foregoing will help you to become expert in diagnosing general symptoms, and whet your appetite for further knowledge and expertise.

Deficient	I (Heart) FULL
II	II 7
III	III 58, IV 3, XII 2 or IV 7, IX 10
IV	IV 3, XII 2 or IV 7, IX 10
V	V 8
VI	VI 5, V 8
VII	VII 37, VIII 4, IX 10
VIII	VIII 4, IX 10
IX	IX 10
X	X 6, IX 10
XI	XI 40, XII 2
XII	XI 12

Deficient	II (Small Intestine) FULL
I	I 5
III	III 58, IV 3, XII 2
IV	IV 3, XII 2
V	V 8, I 5
VI	VI 5, V 8, I 5
VII	VII 37, VIII 4, IX 10, I 5
VIII	VIII 4, IX 10, I 5
IX	IX 10, I 5
X	X 6, IX 10, I 5
XI	XI 40, XII 2, I 5
XII	XII 2, I 5

Deficient	III (Bladder) FULL
I	I 3, IV 4
II	II 7, I 3, IV 4
IV	IV 4

V	V 3, IV 4
VI	VI 5, V 3, IV 4
VII	VII 37, VIII 8, IV 4
VIII	VIII 8, IV 4
IX	IX 10, V 3, IV 4
X	X 6, IX 10, V 3, IV 4
XI	XI 40, XII 1, VIII 8, IV 4
XII	XII 1, VIII 8, IV 4

Deficient	IV (Kidneys) FULL
I	I 3
II	II 7, I 3
III	III 58
V	V 3
VI	VI 5, V 3
VII	VII 37, VIII 8
VIII	VIII 8
IX	IX 10, V 3
X	X 6, IX 10, V 3
XI	XI 40, XII 1, VIII 8
XII	XII 1, VIII 8

Deficient	V (SEX CIRCULATION) FULL
I	I 8
II	II 7, I 8, or II 5
III	III 58, IV 3, XII 2
IV	IV 3, XII 2
VI	VI 5
VII	VII 37, VIII 4, IX 10
VIII	VIII 4, IX 10
IX	IX 10
X	X 6, IX 10
XI	XI 40, XII 2
XII	XII 2

Deficient	VI (Triple-Heater) FULL
I	I 8
II	II 7 or II 5 and I 8
III	III 58, IV 3, XII 2, V 6
IV	IV 3, XII 2, V 6
V	V 6
VII	VII 37, VIII 4, IX 10, V 6
VIII	VIII 4, IX 10, V 6
IX	IX 10, V 6

X	X 6, IX 10, V 6
XI	XI 40, XII 2, V 6
XII	XII 2, V 6

Deficient	VII (GALL BLADDER) FULL
I	I 9, VIII 5
II	II 7, I 9, VIII 5
III	III 58, IV 3, XII 1, VIII 5
IV	IV 3, XII 1, VIII 5
V	V 9, VIII 5
VI	VI 5, V 9, VIII 5
VIII	VIII 5
IX	IX 10, I 9, VIII 5
X	X 6, IX 10, I 9, VIII 5
XI	XI 40, XII 1, VIII 5
XII	XII 1, VIII 5

Deficient	VIII (LIVER) FULL
I	I 9
II	II 7, I 9
III	III 58, IV 3, XII 1
IV	IV 3, XII 1
V	V 9
VI	VI 5, V 9
VII	VII 37
IX	IX 10, I 9
X	X 6, IX 10, I 9
XI	XI 40, XII 1
XII	XII 1

Deficient	IX (LUNGS) FULL
I	I 9, VIII 4
II	II 7, I 9, VIII 4
III	III 58, IV 7
IV	IV 7
V	V 3, IV 7
VI	VI 5, V 3, IV 7
VII	VII 37, VIII 4
VIII	VIII 4
X	X 6
XI	XI 40, XII 1, VIII 4
XII	XII 1, VIII 4

Deficient	X (LARGE INTESTINE) FULL
I	I 9, VIII 4, IX 7
II	II 7, I 9, VIII 4, IX 7
III	III 58, IV 7, IX 7
IV	IV 7, IX 7
V	V 9, VIII 4, IX 7
VI	VI 5, V 9, VIII 4, IX 7
VII	VII 37, VIII 4, IX 7
VIII	VIII 4, IX 7
IX	IX 7
XI	XI 40, XII 1, VIII 4, IX 7
XII	XII 1, VIII 4, IX 7

Deficient	XI (STOMACH) FULL
I	I 3, IV 3, XII 4
II	II 7, I 3, IV 3, XII 4
III	III 58, IV 3, XII 4
IV	IV 3, XII 4
V	V 3, IV 3, XII 4
VI	VI 5, V 3, IV 3, XII 4
VII	VII 37, VIII 4, IX 9, XII 4
VIII	VIII 4, IX 9, XII 4
IX	IX 9, XII 4
X	X 6, IX 9, XII 4
XII	XII 4

Deficient	XII (SPLEEN) FULL
I	I 3, IV 3
II	II 7, I 3, IV 3
III	III 58, IV 3
IV	IV 3
V	V 3, IV 3
VI	VI 5, V 3, IV 3
VII	VII 37, VIII 8, IV 3
VIII	VIII 8, IV 3
IX	IX 9
X	X 6, IX 9.
XI	XI 40

Index